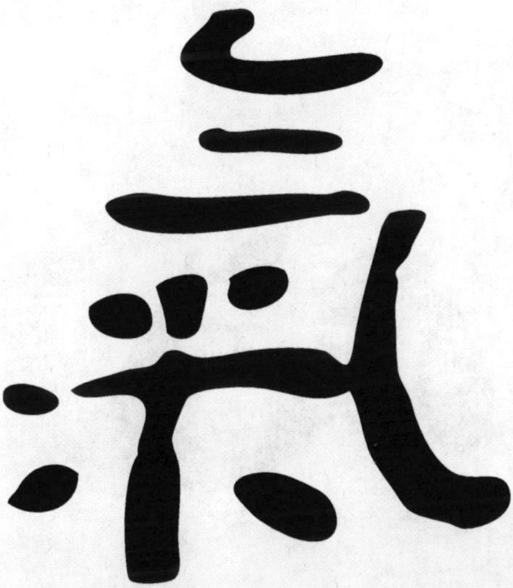

KI (Chi) . . . *Life Force Energy*

Calligraphy by Masato Nakagawa

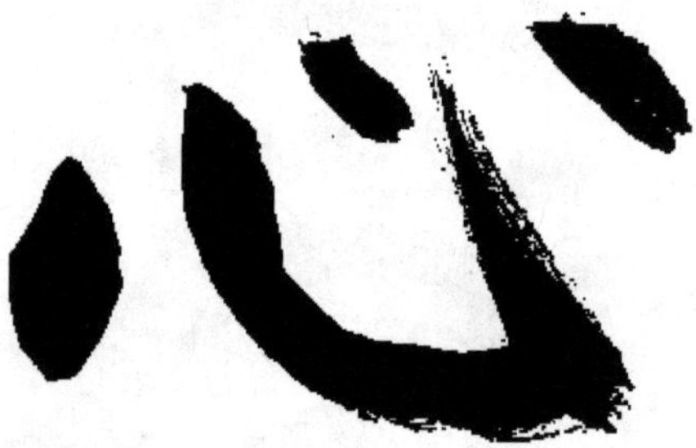

Kokoro . . . Mind / Heart
Calligraphy by Masahiro Oki

Fernando Montoto

Paula Guimarães

Mystery of the Body's Relationship

Kanrenbui

Foreword by Kazuko Tatsumura Hillyer, PhD

KOKORO PUBLISHING

NEW YORK

Kokoro Publishing
20 West 64th Street, #24E
New York City NY 10023
Tel. No. (212) 799-9711
Fax. No. (212) 799-1661
Email: info@gaiahh.com

The exercises and practices in Kanrenbuí are not intended to replace the services of your physician or to provide an alternative to professional medical treatment. Kanrenbuí offers no diagnosis of or treatment for any specific medical problem that you may have. Where it suggests the possible usefulness of certain practices in relation to certain physical problems or mental condition, it does so solely for educational purposes—either to explore the possible relationship of natural breathing to health, or to expose the reader to alternative health and healing approaches.

Printed in the United States

Montoto, Fernando

Kanrenbuí : a arte milenar de cura oriental / Fernando Montoto, Paula Guimarães.
– São Paulo : Oki-Do – Terapia Corporal. 2009.

1. Medicina chinesa 2. Kanrenbuí I. Guimarães, Paula. II. Título. 09-00192 CDD-610.951

Indexes for systemic cataloguing:

1. Kanrenbuí : Medicina chinesa 610.951

ISBN 978-0-9704979-4-9

Designed by Dede Cummings & Daniel Damkoehler
Edited by Ellen Keelan; production by Aleta Alcorn Coursen / dcdesign
Cover art concept by Kazuko Tatsumura Hillyer

The cover design represents the planet earth ("Gaia"), with the top representing blue sky and sunlight, the middle section representing green trees and the brown earth itself, and the red representing the magma beneath the ground.

This edition is printed on recycled, acid-free, paper that meets
the American National Standards Institute z39.48 Standard.

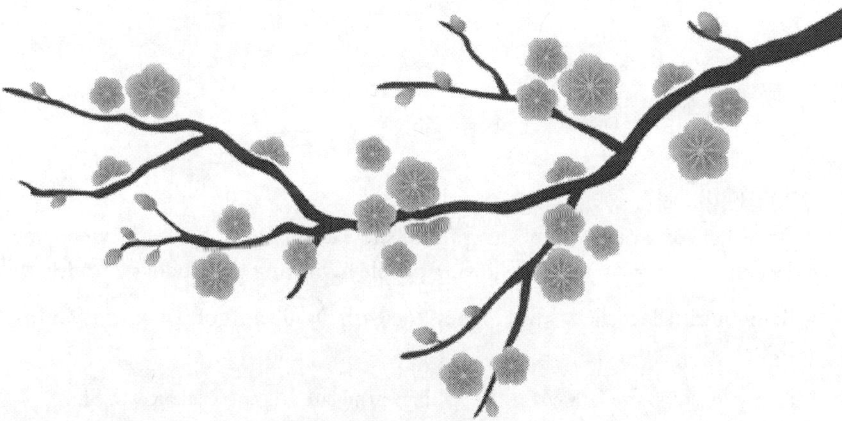

Our thanks to Masahiro Oki taught us a path.

Acknowledgments

On behalf of Kokoro Publishing's Holistic Health Book Series, I extend my deepest appreciation to the following people in making these books a reality:

To my spiritual teachers: His Holiness the 14th Dalai Lama of Tibet and Mother Theresa.

To my masters: the late Masahiro Oki and the late Masato Nakagawa, Sr.

To Reimi Takeuchi for assisting me in translating the book.

To Soushisha Co., Ltd and the president Haruo Kitani for their generosity in allowing us publish this translated version in the U.S.

To Mie Kadokuchi, the illustrator, for allowing us to use her original drawings in this English version.

To Dede Cummings and her staff at DCDesign for their dedication to our book publishing projects.

Gasshou

With deepest gratitude, Kazuko Tatsumura OMD, PhD., May 2009

Preface

by Kazuko Tatsumura Hillyer, OMD, Ph.D.

Osamu Tatsumura is my younger brother, and at the same time he is my teacher. Through him, I have learned much of the teaching of the late, legendary Master Masahiro Oki.

After Master Oki's passing, Osamu Tatsumura, as the closest and longest disciple of master Oki, eventually became the leader of Okido Yoga and further developed its unique techniques. Today, my brother is admired as the most important teacher in the field of holistic healing in Japan, traveling all over the world to teach and give lectures. His book *Deep Breath Changes Your Body and Mind/Sprit* is already a force in Japan, and just published in the United States by Kokoro Publishing in 2008.

Fernando Montoto and Paula Guimarães both studied with Sensei Oki, and their work reflects the teachings of the master. I'm very happy that Kokoro Publishing's new book, *Mystery of the Body's Relationship: Kanrenbui*, is now being published in the United States and we celebrate the work of this team of practicioners. I'm sure it will benefit many people throughout the world.

This book is the fourth in a series of nine books on health and spirituality being published by Kokoro Publishing. The series includes the following titles:

- *Overcoming Cancer and Other Difficult Diseases in a Holistic Way*, by Tomeko Mitsui and Kazuko Tatsumura Hillyer (published in 2003, second edition in 2007)

- *Your Immune Revolution* and *Healing Your Healing Power*, by Toru Abo & Kazuko Tatsumura Hillyer (published in 2007)
- *Deep Breath Changes Your Body and Mind/Spirit*, by Osamu Tatsumura (published in 2008)
- *Mystery of the Body's Relationship: Kanrenbui*, by Fernando and Paula Montoto
- *Joy of Yoga*, by Masahiro Oki (scheduled for release in 2009)

I hope you will enjoy these books, and please send us comments. Contact Gaia Holistic Health at *www.gaiahh.com* or (212) 799-9711 or *kazuko@gaiahh.com* for more information about upcoming books and how to purchase them.

Contents

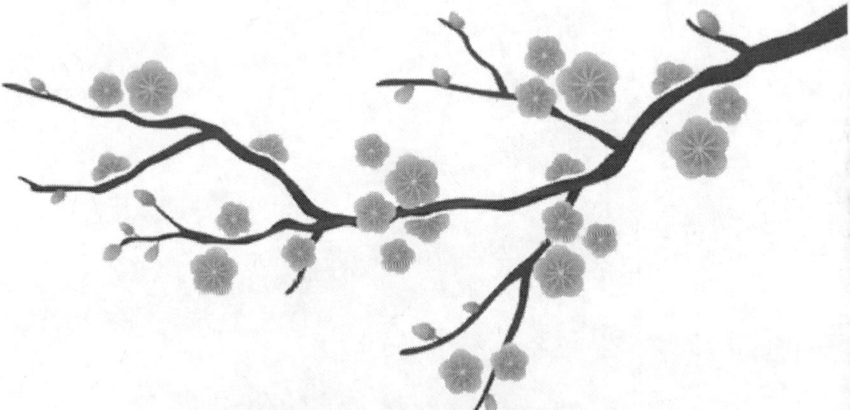

Mystery of the Body's Relationship

Kanrenbui

Introduction

One day, a student asked a sensei (teacher, in Japanese), who was a master in kanrenbui, how these studies began. The sensei explained that among the ancient people of Japan, there were older people who lived in isolated regions in the mountains. They watched nature and meditated on it, analyzing the relationship that the wild animal established with its own body. Kanrenbui was born from these observations.

KANRENBUI is a study with millenary records in oriental medicine, but it was in Japan that it was developed and expanded. Up until today, thestudy of kanrenbui is passed on from father to son, from teacher to student, from generation to generation, as is typical of the ancient traditions.

In the philosophy of the Far East, the harmonious and balanced flow of vital energy is fundamental to the health of the individual. This energy is called ki by the Japanese and chi by the Chinese, similar to the prana of the Indians.

We had the opportunity to live and study in Oki Yoga Dojo, in Mishima, Japan, the school of Masahiro Oki. Oki sensei, as he was called, was a master of several techniques to develop human potential, such as yoga, oriental medicine and martial arts. Among these is kanrenbui, which can be described as the related points in the body, since it is the study of the interrelationships of parts of the body.

According to Masahiro Oki, nature and the human being are governed by a natural process of change, equilibrium and stability. When this process is interrupted, whether due to physical, emotional or psychic blocks, the body manifests a pain or symptom. With the technical intervention of kanrenbui, one can restore the good flow of this natural process.

This method conceives the human body as integrated in many relationships. When we feel a pain or adverse symptom, we look for certain areas and points related to these discomforts. By repeatedly pressure on these points, we notice a radical change in these feelings.

In kanrenbui, the symmetry of the physical body is very important, as is the case in every oriental cure art, like yoga, tai chi chuan and martial arts in general. If we consider the physical body, the mind and flow of live as a whole, we should associate pains and symptoms not only to the physical part, but also to its relation with changes in thoughts and habits.

With kanrenbui, we learn that when a person has a pain, postural imbalance or limitation in physical movement, on pressing certain vital points, we unblock the flow of ki (internal energy), thus improving the physical, organic state, allowing for a deeper breathing and increasing physical flexibility that, in turn, is related to mental flexibility.

Each part of our physical body (foot, hand, ear, eyes, top of the head), corresponds to the whole body. They are like maps of the human physical structure. Thus, we can use one of these several parts to treat the totality of the body, as we will see in Figures I.1, I.2 and I.3 below from ancient oriental medicine.

According to this method, when we feel a pain or an area is tense, we must identify the points related to this body zone and press them at least 20 times. It is however important that this pressure is accompanied by breathing. This is an essential item for the change and reestablishment of ki harmony.

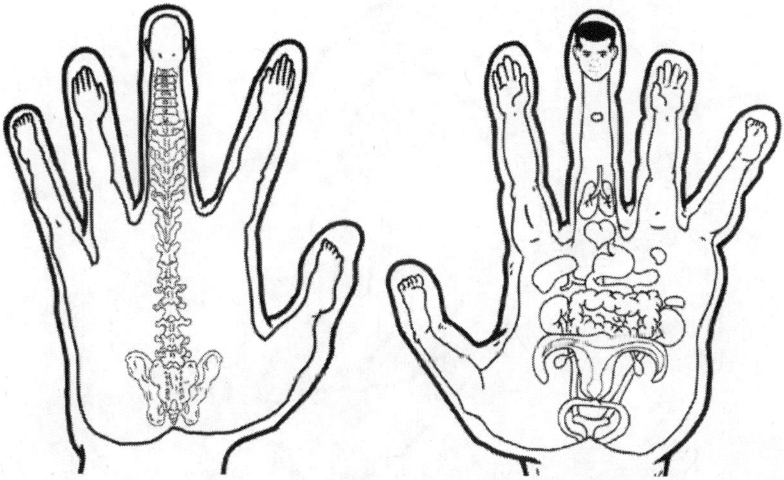

Figure I.1 In the hands we find relationships with the whole body

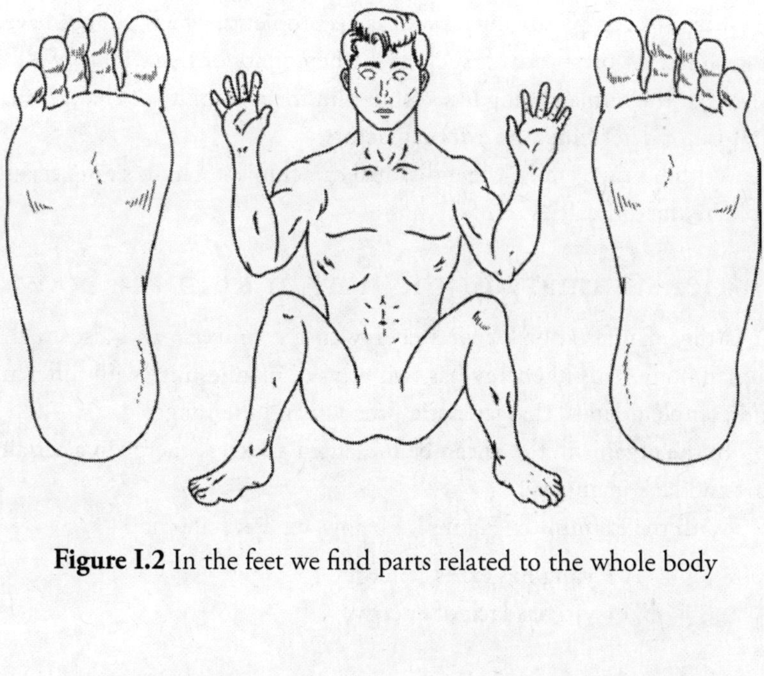

Figure I.2 In the feet we find parts related to the whole body

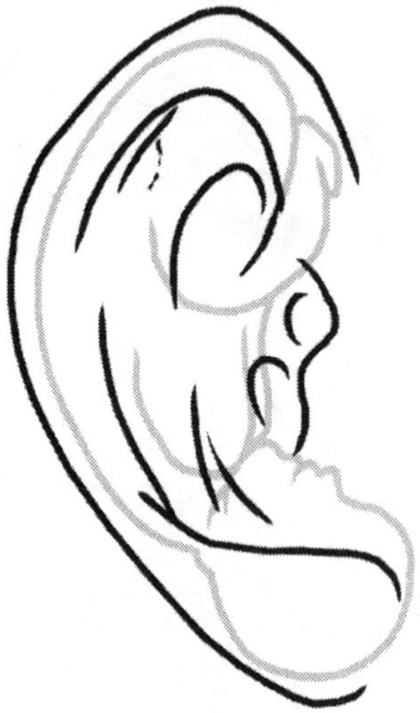

Figure I.3 There is a representation of the body in the fetal position in the ear

Man is a complex being, as well as his problems, which can be viewed from different perspectives, such as the hereditary or behavioral. We believe that the human being has within him the possibility of change, that is, it is not determined by external factors.

With his own effort, the individual can connect with his essence and lapidate the difficulties of life.

Brief summary of the flow of **ki** in the body

Ki is the manifestation of vital energy in the universe and also in the human body. This ki energy has two ways of manifesting, with different and complementary characteristics: the yin and the yang.

In the organism, the ki can be presented as excess energy in a certain part and lack in another.

With the example of Figure I.4 below, we can state that:

A = yang has excess energy
B = yin has lack of energy.

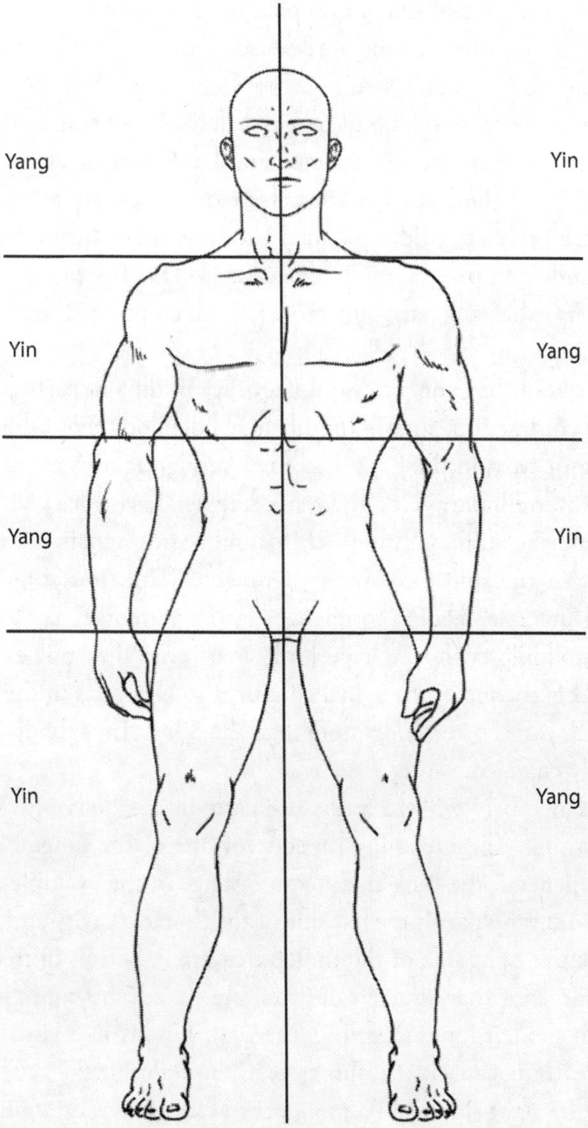

Figure I.4 The yin and yang forces act in zigzag in the body

When there is a blocking or a pain in an A yang area, this blocking is manifested in other A yang areas. Also, if the blocking is in the B yin area, it may also be manifested in other B yin areas.

The yang parts in the body are characterized by being full of energy; they are stiffer, tense, hot, contracted and have more acute pains. While the yin parts of the body are characterized by lack of energy; they are more flaccid, relaxed, cold, expanded and have more diffuse pains.

Yin and yang work as complementary forces. The tenser, stiffer and full of energy the yang parts, the more flaccid, empty and short of energy the yin parts.

Stiffness in the yang parts and flaccidity in the yin parts can change muscular contraction, interfering in the whole body. For example: if in the posterior part, in the back, there is a very great stiffness on one side of the paravertebral muscles, the other side will have a flaccidity (yin) to compensate the stiffness (yang). If this imbalance remains, it can result in change in the spinal column's alignment. With time, this misalignment can increase, leading to changes in the vertebrae, and potentially causing scoliosis, cyphosis, hyperlordosis or even disk bulges and disk hernias. This change in the spinal column also interferes in the hip position, which can shorten a leg more than the other. Thus, body posture is completely changed.

Imbalance between yin and yang parts in the body also interferes with breathing. The breathing capacity of one of the lungs is compromised: in general, the lung that is more yang. In the example in Figure I.4, the more yang part is the left side of the thoracic cavity and the more yin part is the right side of the thoracic cavity. A person in this organic state will probably have the left nostril more closed, showing a yang contraction in the left lung; therefore, the right lung is in a yin state, with greater breathing capacity. In this case, in the abdominal

part, the right side will be more contracted, in a yang state, and the left side more expanded, in a yin state.

With this energy and physical state, the person can have distortions in the thoracic cavity, in the hip and length of the arms and legs.

There is a complex network of blood vessels, arteries and veins essential to our life in our body. When a region in the body has a muscular contraction, or excess energy in an internal organ (yang), and in another there is lack of energy (yin), circulation is compromised in this region and also in the regions related to it. The blood flow in the arteries and venous return find difficulties due to the tension, stiffness and even flaccidity in regions of the body. Therefore, imbalance of the yin and yang in the body also change the blood flow.

As we have seen, imbalance of the yin and yang interferences in the body posture, functioning of the internal organs, breathing, blood circulation; all these factors interference in the vital force, in the ki, in the person's energy.

In this state, each action practiced by the person will demand from him/her greater energy use, both physical and mental, because the body produces a certain effort to try and compensate for the imbalances. The person suffers more with these imbalances. Even if they do not manifest as diseases, there is a spending of energy to achieve its objectives.

The ancestral diagnosis of the body

Let us look at another way of relating the body within kanrenbui. This is a very ancient form that was used in the Orient to diagnose the body. We will divide the body into three parts:

A = Upper part of the body = Head
B = Middle part of the body = Torso
C = Lower part of the body = Legs

We will also divide the arms and legs into four parts: A, B, C and D, as shown in Figure I.5 below.

A disorder, pain or imbalance in part A can be treated in another part A. If there is a disorder in part B, we will treat the other B parts, and likewise for part C and D. In most cases, it is more efficient to treat the parts related to the symptom than only the region where it is presented.

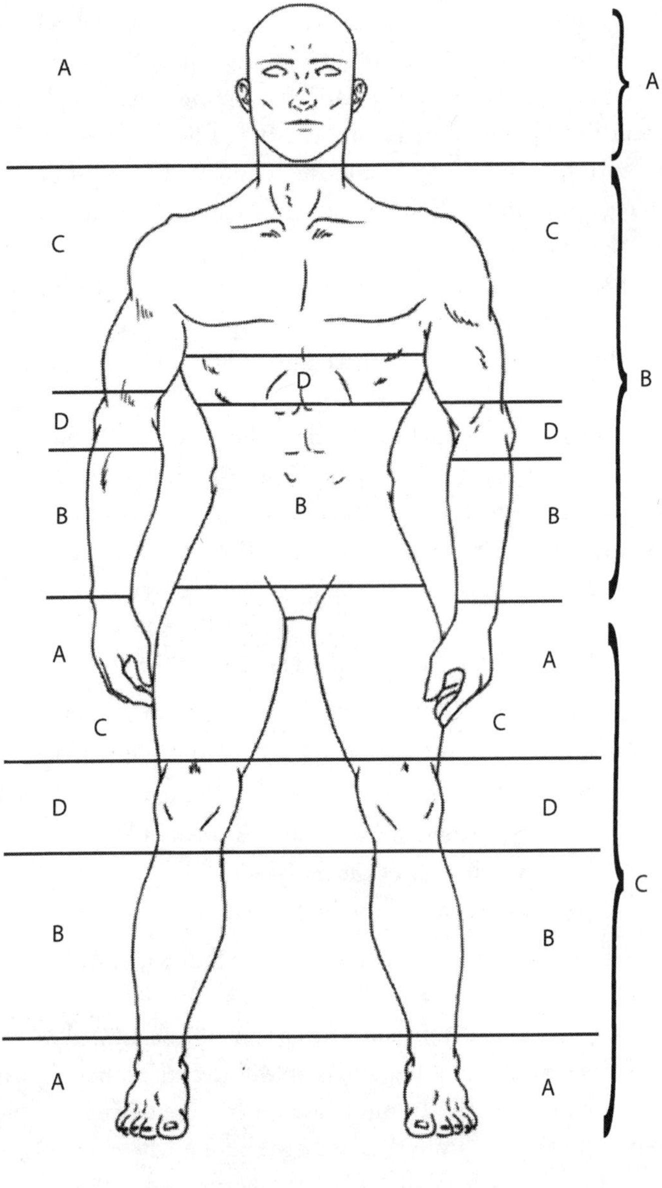

Figure I.5 The ancient form of diagnosing the body in the Orient

Part A: Extremities of the body, head, hands and feet

The head is related to the hands and feet. This means that we can treat in the hands and feet a headache or any other symptom in the face. The extremities are interrelated. For example, when we massage the hands and/or feet, there is a deep relaxation in the mind. We can make a full massage of the feet in a person who is experiencing an anxiety crisis, for example. This will soon calm the person and cause a mental relaxation. Meanwhile, when we wish to be more awake, with the mind more active and open to new learning or when our mind is tired, dull, sleepy and must wake p to some mental activity (study, take a test, give a lecture, write a text), we must massage the back of the hands strongly, for some minutes, pressing the points between the bones, the metacarpus with the thumbs. We will immediately feel more awake and with greater clarity of reasoning.

The neck is related to the wrists and ankles. To loosen a stiffness in the neck, head or a tension in the cervix, we can loosen the wrists and ankles with circulation motions, stretching and massages.

Part B: Lower part of the abdomen, arms and legs

The regions of the small intestine and large intestine, the forearms and the lower part of the legs are interrelated. To improve the functioning of the intestines, we can stimulate the points in the inner region of the forearms. Intestinal functioning also improves when we stimulate the legs with a walk. Varices and poor circulation in the legs indicate an intestinal malfunctioning. To improve blood circulation in the legs, one must improve the intestine's condition.

Part C: Upper part of the body, arms and legs

The region of the shoulders and trapezius, the thoracic cavity and upper part of the legs and arms are interrelated. For example: for greater flexibility of the movement in opening the legs, we can press the part anterior in the inner side of the arms, near the armpits, which relaxes the legs, facilitating its opening movement. In the upper part of the arms, there are several points to treat tension in the trapezius. These points are very efficient in treating stiff necks and strong pains in the trapezius and will be taught in chapter 6 referring to the arms.

Part D: Middle part of the abdomen, arms and legs

The middle part of the arms and legs is related to the middle part of the abdomen, digestive and gastric organs. As example, we can mention a pain in the knee, which can indicate an imbalance in the stomach or liver. This imbalance can be treated in points in the median region of the arms, near the elbow. The knee will also improve as the organic imbalance improves.

Based on our clinical experience, we can state that, for an effective and long-lasting improvement of the knee, the treatment should not be limited to this part of the body; one must balance the middle organs of the abdomen.

It is very common to find people with pains and inflammations in the tendons or elbow joint. Diagnosis by touching the abdomen reveals an imbalance in the liver or gallbladder. On treating the liver imbalance, the pain and inflammation in the arm disappear, but if we treat the inflammation spot only, we will hardly be successful.

1

The abdomen

Oriental medicine states that the well-being of the internal organs (stomach, spleen, pancreas, gallbladder, intestines, liver, bladder and kidneys) is of fundamental importance to the balance of ki.

Ki, in the hermeneutic tradition of the Far East, is the vital force. This signifier – ki – appears in Japanese language under several forms, but always related to the healthy or the sick. For example, a pleasant thing is kimochi; or, when the person is sick, he/she is bioki.

The changes in the flow of ki in the body (excess or lack) cause diseases. We can map the ki in the body of the person, identifying when it is in excess – jitsu – or when it is empty – kyo. This can be diagnosed in several ways: through the wrist, posture and internal organs, which is the form used in the Oki-Do method, to be presented herein.

When the ki is altered, the organs become hard and tense, which in turn modifies the physical posture. For example, when the internal organs are tenser on one side than on the other, they change the position of the pelvis, making one leg shorter than the other, which in turn will change the position of the spinal vertebrae.

Breathing is a structuring factor in the well-being of the individual. For some medicines from the Orient, like the Indian (*ayurveda*), breathing is fundamental for the balance of vital energy. The *prana*, to the Indians, is a combination of movements with breathing. The poses of Indian *yoga*, the paths of martial arts and techniques like *chi-kung* and *tai chi* use this combination of movement with breathing. In *kanrenbui,* it is important to reconcile breathing with the movement of pressure, for both the therapist applying the treatment and the one who receives it.

When we press the points related to the internal organs that are altered, it is usual to notice that the breathing of the person who receives the treatment becomes deeper. The organ immediately becomes more balanced and free from its tensions, providing

a more harmonious state in the body and a deeper breathing. This causes the posture to be more erect and adequate and the mind to be more peaceful.

If we analyze deep breathing, we notice that the organs expand when we breathe in and contract when we breathe out. The autonomic nervous system, formed by the sympathetic and parasympathetic nervous systems, is stimulated with this dynamics and the whole body becomes more balanced.

Let us look at an example of how the whole body is connected (holistic relation) and how an affected organ can create a general disturbance in the body, disturbing breathing and posture. When the organs on the right side are tense, that is, the liver and gallbladder are in a jitsu state (stiff), we note that breathing is altered, since the lung on the same side works with limitation due to being in a kyo state, with lack of energy. This can be noticed in the right nostril, which has a smaller orifice. The right leg also becomes tenser and usually shorter.

According to Chinese medicine, emotions have direct relation to the internal organs. Each organ represents a feeling. The liver is related to anger. Notice that when a person has a lot of anger inside him/her, his/her right side is usually tenser and the right shoulder is projected forward. Therefore, through the posture, we diagnose the organic functioning: if the organs are kyo (empty) or jitsu (full).

Many muscular pains in the spine and inflammations are the result of organic malfunctioning. In this chapter, we will show the main points related specifically to the internal organs in the abdomen. These points serve to harmonize the tanden, the physical and energy center of the body, located in the lower part of the abdomen.

Each point should be pressed at least 20 times with the flesh of the thumb. For a more effective treatment, breathe out with each pressure, this applying to both therapist and person receiving the treatment.

For didactic purposes, we divided the study of the internal organs, relating them with the parts of the abdomen:

- upper part
- central part
- median part
- lateral part
- lower part

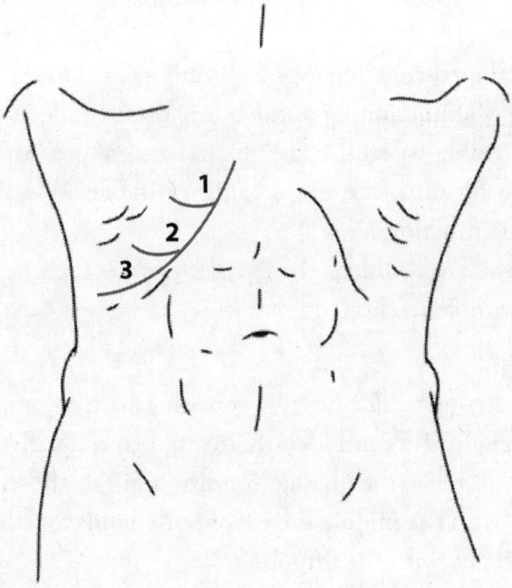

Figure 1.1 Region of the liver and gallbladder

Upper part of the abdomen
Right side

The right side of the abdomen, below the ribs, is the region where we can locate the liver and the gallbladder (see Figure 1.1).

Part 1 is more related to the gallbladder, and parts 2 and 3 with the liver. This right side of the top part of the abdomen is related to the neck, as we can see in Figure 1.2. However, one important caution must be taken: the technique of pressing points in the neck must be restricted to the inner part of the sternocleidomastoid muscle, since this region is very sensitive and the person may not have the desired result.

Several symptoms are related to the tension we can find in the liver and gallbladder:

- anger;
- stiffness in the tendons and tendonitis;
- pain in the nape, neck and cervix;
- malfunctioning of the bowel.

In oriental medicine, the liver is directly related to the tendons, neck and to anger. Malfunctioning of the bowel directly affects the liver, since the body is unable to release the toxins, and one of the functions of the liver is to disintoxicate the organism. The accumulation of toxins retained by malfunctioning

of the bowel overburdens the liver. Therefore, for a healthy liver, the bowel must work at least once a day.

Diagnosis

The first step is to diagnose by touching with the fingers points 1, 2 and 3 (see Figure 1.1) and identify the part that is stiffer or with pain. The touch to diagnose the organic condition in the abdomen should always be done with the middle fingers of both hands together. We do not press the abdomen with the thumbs.

Treatment

Look in the neck for a point in the region related to the point to be treated in the abdomen (see Figure 1.2). Press at least 20 times, always on breathing out. This treatment should be applied with the person lying down with the abdomen facing up, so that the neck muscles are relaxed, especially the sternocleidomastoid muscle.

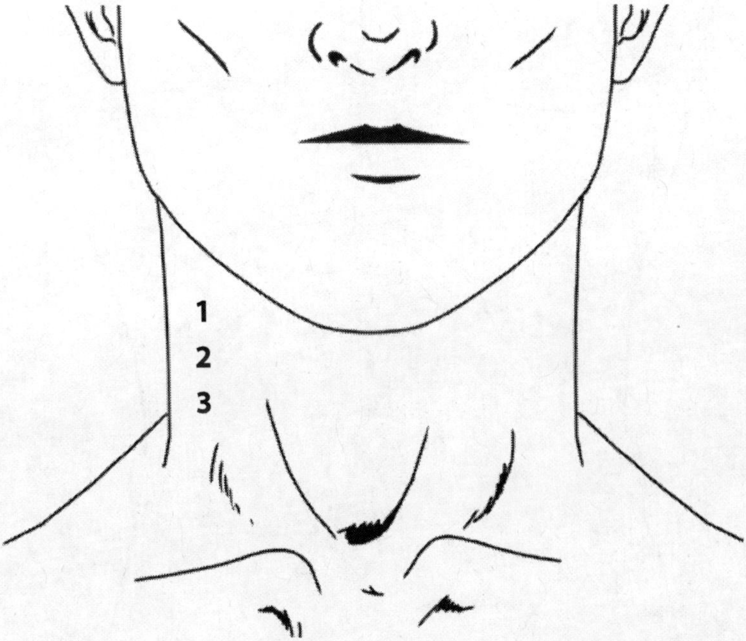

Figure 1.2 Points related to the liver and gallblander.

Left side

The stomach, spleen and pancreas are located on the top part of the left side of abdomen, below the ribs.

Parts 4 and 5 are related to the stomach. In general, very nervous and worried people have pains in this region.

Part 6 is related to the spleen and pancreas. They are very efficient points in the treatment of diabetics and people who eat a lot of sugar and sweets (see Figure 1.3).

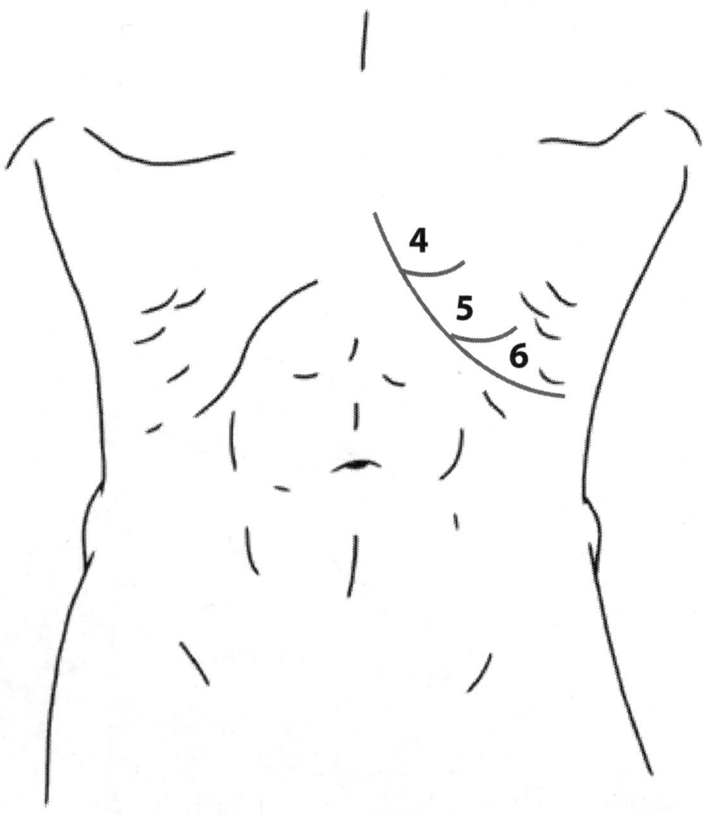

Figure 1.3 Region of the stomach, spleen and pancreas

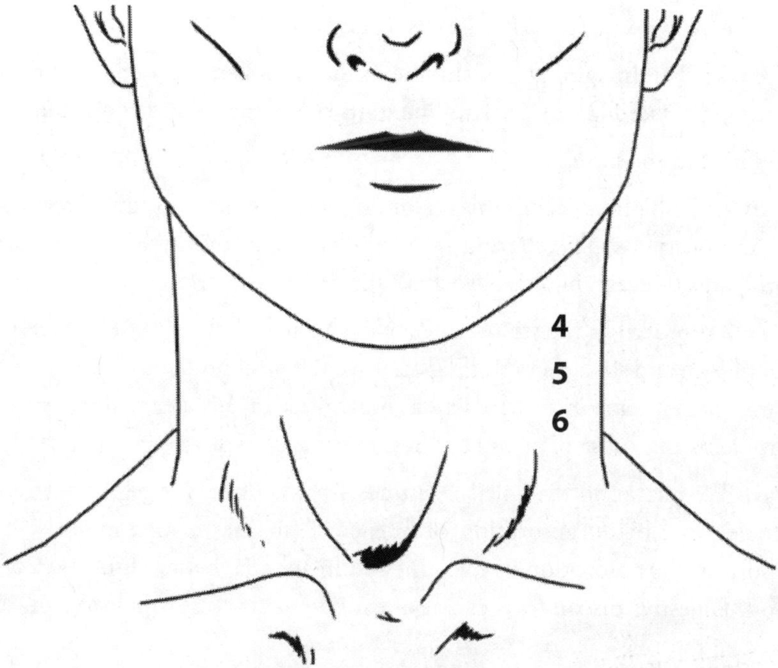

Figure 1.4 Points related to the stomach, spleen and pancreas

Several symptoms are related to the tension we can find in the stomach, spleen and pancreas:

- indigestion;
- heartburn;
- gastritis;
- stomach ulcers;
- diabetes;
- worry and mental tension.

The same technique should be used on this side, with diagnosis in the abdomen and treatment on the left side of the neck, according to Figure 1.4.

Central part of the abdomen

We traced an imaginary median line in the abdomen and divided it into three parts (see Figure1.5). This line starts below the sternum and continues toward the navel.

Part 1, the highest part of this region, right below the sternum, is related to the heart. People suffering from hypertension, dysrhythmia, cardiac problems or even anguish have great stiffness in this region.

Part 2 is related to the stomach. People who are constantly stressed feel a lot of pain and stiffness in this region. Psychological problems like depression, mental tension and anxiety also manifest in this area. All digestive problems can cause pain and stiffness in these points.

Part 3 is related to the small intestine. Treatment of this region is very efficient for better absorption of nutrients. In cases of osteoporosis, it improves the absorption of calcium, and in anemia, better absorption of iron. Digestive discomforts can also manifest as stiffness in this region.

Diagnosis

Press the median line in the center of the abdomen and feel, through a slow and deep touch, the most painful or stiff point in this region (see Figure 1.5).

Treatment

Seek the point related to the abdomen in the median line on the top of the head (see Figure 1.6). Press this point until you obtain slight relief in the pain caused by the pressure in the point or, at least, 20 times, always accompanying the breathing. With this type of treatment, breathing becomes deeper, causing the person to become calmer. The result will be a relief in the stiffness previously found in the abdominal region.

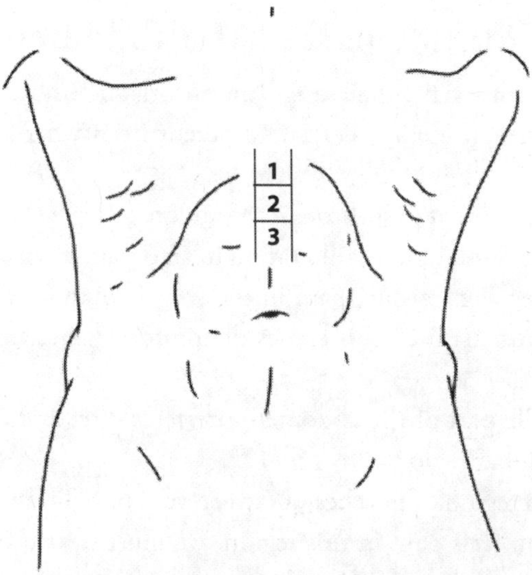

Figure 1.5 Central part of the abdomen

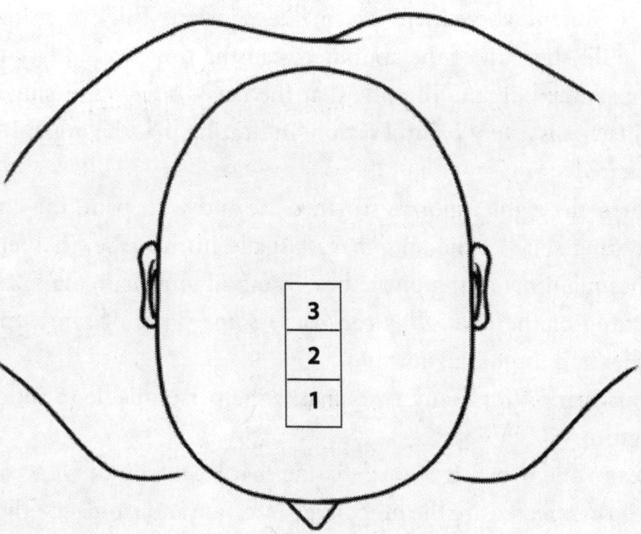

Figure 1.6 Points related to the central part of the abdomen in the head

Middle part of the abdomen

Back pains mostly have their origin in an organic imbalance. This is a concept of oriental medicine, quite different from what is conceived in the Occident.

All the nerves that pass through the abdomen have their origin in the spinal column. When there is alteration in an organ, it will cause interference in the nerving, causing pain in the spinal column, in turn altering the lumbar musculature. This causes discomfort, which can often cause lumbar pains.

The middle part of the abdomen interferes directly in the musculature of the lumbar region and

in the end region of the chest, between vertebrae T8 and T12. Whenever the person feels pain in this region, we must treat the jitsu parts in the center of the abdomen in its related points. This region can be treated on the top of the head.

We start by checking the position of the navel: if it is facing down, to the left or right. The direction of the navel reveals the most dilated part of the abdomen, where there is a small expansion. This expansion in the organs pulls the skin of the abdomen, causing the navel to face the side of the expanded organ. The side that the navel is facing usually has too much jitsu. It is a very painful region, indicating that the organ is dilated and irritated.

When the right region is stiffer, tense and with pain, this indicates a more yang state of the abdomen. Usually in this case, the person already has malfunctioning of the bowel, modifying, as we have seen, the functioning of the liver. This can cause some types of symptoms, like headaches and lumbar pains.

Constipation for many years makes the person liable to suffer from rheumatism.

Meanwhile, when it is the left side that is stiffer and with pain, the organs most affected are the lung, large intestine and stomach. The stomach is an organ connected directly with the psychological side, which can revert into intense pains in the lumbar.

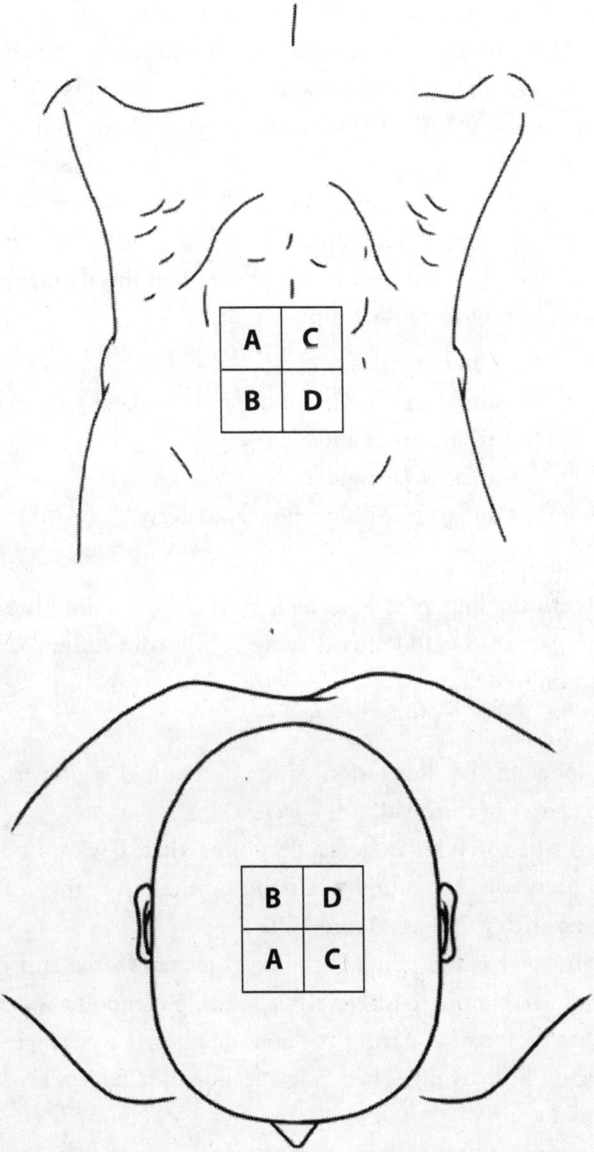

Figure 1.7 Middle part of the abdomen and its related points in the head

When the person faces stressful situations and difficulty to accept facts – difficulty to *digest* the happenings, so to speak – the chest closes, the thoracic cavity becomes more contracted, breathing becomes shorter, causing imbalance in the functions of the sympathetic and parasympathetic nervous system, altering the stomach and, consequently, digestion. In oriental medicine, this condition is called *stomach prolapse,* or commonly: fallen stomach. The fall of the stomach presses the organs from the left side, causing pains in the central region of the abdomen.

This condition can cause symptoms like:

- lumbar pains;
- drop of the immune system, becoming vulnerable to flu, colds and allergies;
- menstrual cramps;
- inflammation of the sciatic nerve.

Diagnosis

Press with the fingers of both hands the points around the navel, in the central part of the abdomen, trying to find the stiffest part and/or part with pain (see Figure 1.7).

Treatment

Each letter in the illustration of the abdominal region has its corresponding letter in the head.

With the person lying in dorsal decubitus, that is, with the abdomen facing up, press with the thumb the point on the top of the head related to the region with pain (see Figure 1.7).

We can see that the point of the head related to the stiff quadrant of the abdomen is more sensitive. After pressing this point several times, we note that the median part of the abdomen starts to change, relaxing the stiff region little by little, bringing a feeling of relief from the pain on being pressed again.

This treatment brings immediate relief to the stiff region in the abdomen and treats all symptoms resulting from the tension present in the organs, such as a change in the digestive part, relief of the lumbar pains and of the sciatic nerve, among others.

Lateral part of the abdomen

These parts correspond to the area that goes from the end of the ribs up to the iliac crest. This region is related to the large intestine.

Pains, tensions or stiffness in this lateral part of the abdomen can cause alterations in the arm on the same side, like inflammations in the wrist, elbow, tendonitis, poor circulation.

As shown in Figure 1.9, the lateral regions of the abdomen are related to the areas of the anterior part of the forearm.

Diagnosis

With the fingers of both hands together, press the sides of the abdomen and find the stiffest point of one side and the other (see Figure 1.8).

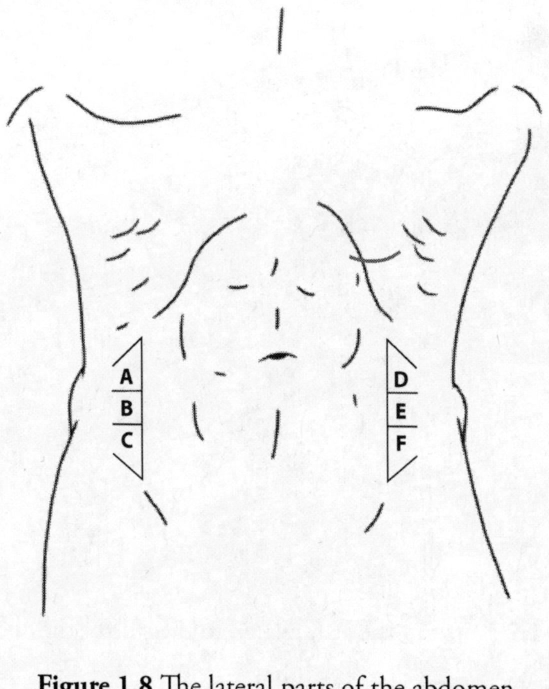

Figure 1.8 The lateral parts of the abdomen

Treatment

Still with the person lying down, place the arms by the body, with the palms of the hands facing up, on the same side in which there is stiffness or discomfort in the abdomen. Find in the forearm a sensitive point, which should be located at the same height as the pain in the abdomen. Trace an imaginary line from the painful region in the abdomen up to the forearm, and you will thus find the point to be treated. Press the point with the thumb and massage it with the palm of the hand (see Figure 1.9).

When we combine the treatment of this area with the anterior (center of the abdomen), we obtain many benefits to the internal organs: a feeling of comfort, relief from back pains and deeper breathing.

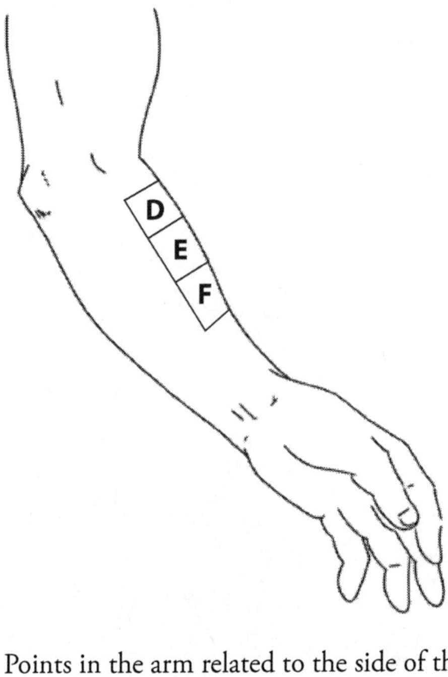

Figure 1.9 Points in the arm related to the side of the abdomen

Lower part of the abdomen

The lower part of the abdomen, between the iliac bones of the pelvis, on the right and left side, is related, respectively, to the right and left legs.

The pain or stiffness in this region can cause alterations in the leg of the same side, for example, pains in the knee and ankle joints, swelling in the leg, pains in the posterior part of the leg, poor circulation and varices.

All these symptoms can be improved if we treat the points related to this region, relieving the stiffness or pain in the abdomen.

When a person has pain in the knee, groin, ankle or in another part of the leg, we must always check this region below the abdomen.

We will certainly find a strong pain in this region, on the same side of the leg. We will make a mistake if we treat only the location of the pain itself, which can cause only a momentary relief. For a more effective treatment, before treating the location of the pain, we must treat the region below the abdomen in its related points, in the head.

According to Figure 1.10, parts A and G are related to the large intestine.

Parts B, C, E, F are related to the ovaries and uterus in women.

Part D is related to the bladder and prostate. The point related to this region on the top of the head treats cystitis, urinary infection, inflammation in the bladder and disorders in the prostate.

Diagnosis

With the person lying down in dorsal decubitus, that is, with the abdomen facing up, first check which side of the lower abdominal region suffers the most pain. Also check the angle of the foot in relation to the bed or the floor. The foot must be at an angle of 60 degrees in relation to the floor (see Figure 1.11). If it is "fallen", that is, with less than 60 degrees, it means that the pelvis is bent to one side, affecting the balance of the internal organs. While in cases where the foot is at 90 degrees in relation to the floor, we interpret that the organs on the same side are tense and stiff and the hip very closed.

The position of the feet indicates the position of the pelvis. When

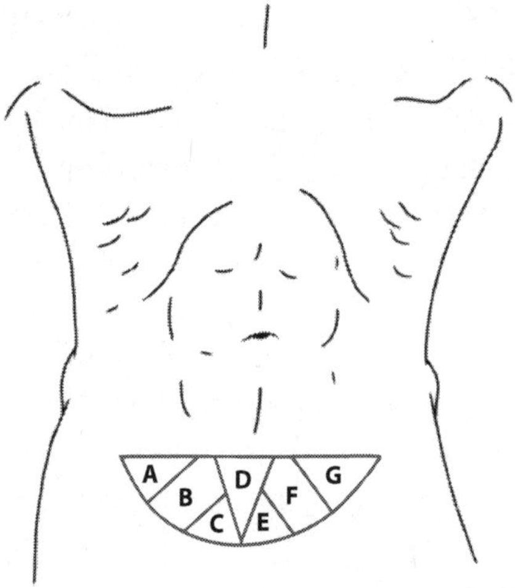

Figure 1.10 Lower part of the abdomen

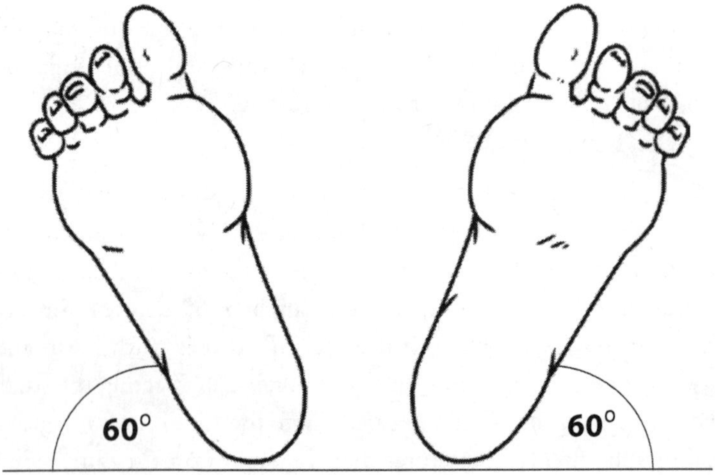

Figure 1.11 Ideal position of the feet

the pelvis is bent, the person can have symptoms like: menstrual cramps, pains in the knee (due to forcing a joint more than another) and lumbar pains.

Treatment

With the person lying down with the abdomen facing up, look in the head for the point related to the lower area of the abdomen and that has pain or stiffness.

Press the point with the thumb several times (see Figure 1.12).

If the pain in the abdominal region is in part B or F (see Figure 1.10), also press, as an extra point, the points in the anterior part of the thigh, right above the knee, on the same side of the abdominal pain (see Figure 1.13). This pressure can be done with the thumb and with the palm of the hand.

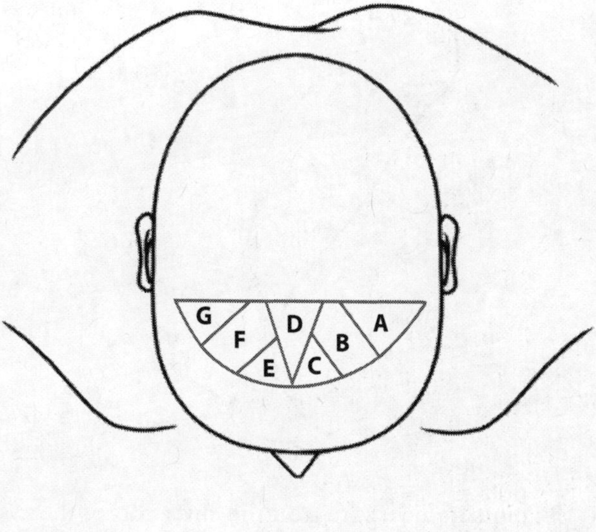

Figure 1.12 Points in the head related to the lower part of the abdomen

If the pain in the abdominal region is located in parts C and E (see Figure 1.10), the region to be treated will be in the anterior part of the thigh, very near the groin, on the same side of the abdominal pain. The pressure can be done with the thumb or with the palm of the hand. This point treats the uterus, ovaries and prostate (see Figure 1.13).

Through the Kanrenbui method, it is considered to be a sign of health when, once diagnosed and treated, the person does not have any kind of pain in the abdominal region. This shows that the person has harmonic energy and that the center of the tanden is in equilibrium.

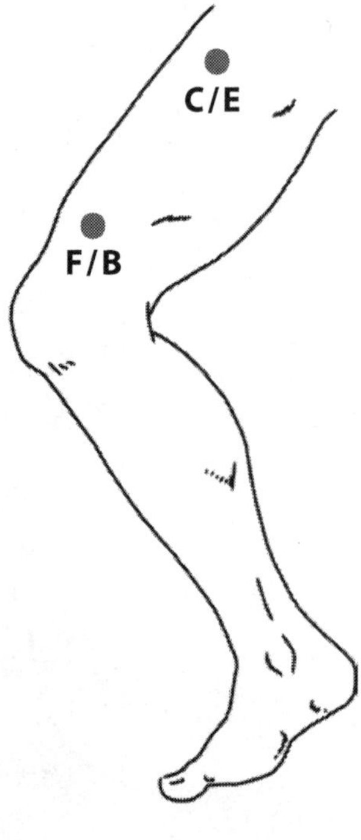

Figure 1.13 Points in the legs to treat the lower part of the abdomen

Large intestine

The large intestine is the organ responsible for eliminating feces; it is also where liquids needed by the body are processed and absorbed. It is therefore important that it works at least once a day. Even thus, we accumulate residues from previous feces, called shokuben, which remain deposited in the intestinal loops.

Our body is made up of 60% of liquids. A great part of this liquid is absorbed in the large intestine. When we accumulate previous feces in our intestine, they release several types of toxins, which are absorbed together with the water and taken to the whole body. Therefore, constipation indicates an intoxicated organism.

Oriental medicine considers it very important that the bowel works one or twice a day, depending on the amount of foods ingested, since a clean bowel indicates clean blood, free of toxins. According to this oriental concept, good quality of the blood is associated with good functioning of the bowel and, consequently, good health.

Each part of the intestine is related to a part of the body, as shown in Figure 1.14. Therefore, the deposit of shokuben in the intestine causes an alteration in it, which can become an inflammation in the location where it is found and also affect the related part in the body.

The entire contour of the head is related to the large intestine, therefore it is in this contour that we treat the organ, as shown in Figure 1.15.

Diagnosis

One of the ways of diagnosing the intestine can be as follows: hit the contour of the head gently with the hand closed, checking where the sound is graver or more acute. The region where the sound is graver is usually the most sensitive and, oftentimes, painful.

Treatment

Press this more sensitive region with the thumb until there is a relief of the pain in this point of the head. Thus, you will be treating the region related to the large intestine, as shown in Figure 1.15.

In case of people with constipation problems, it is very important to press the entire contour of the head.

Many symptoms, like headaches, rheumatisms and itching of the scalp are associated with malfunctioning of the intestine.

When the person suffers from rheumatoid arthritis, popularly known as rheumatism, the first thing we must do is ask about his/her bowel functioning. Next, we must diagnose the abdominal region by touching and treat the intestine in its related points, located in the head according to Figure 1.15.

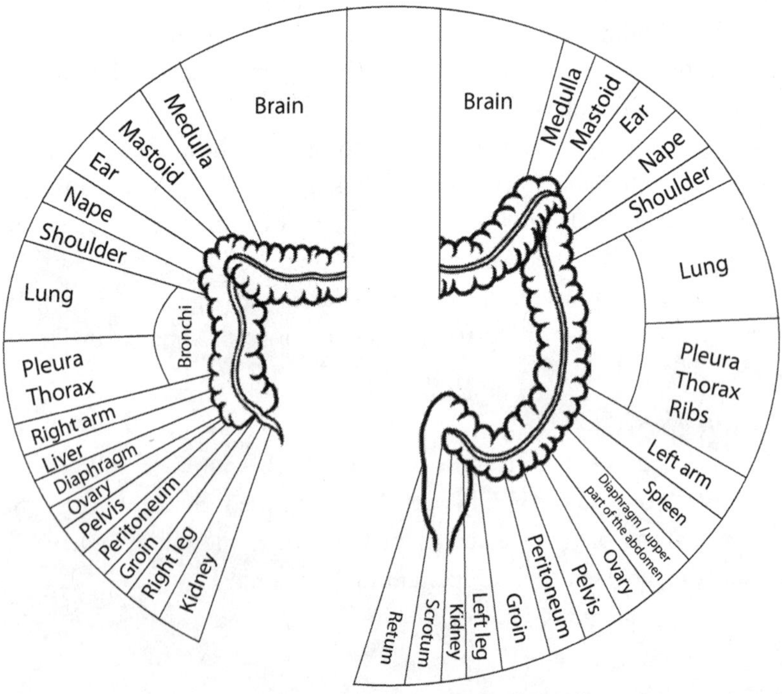

Figure 1.14 Relations of the large intestine

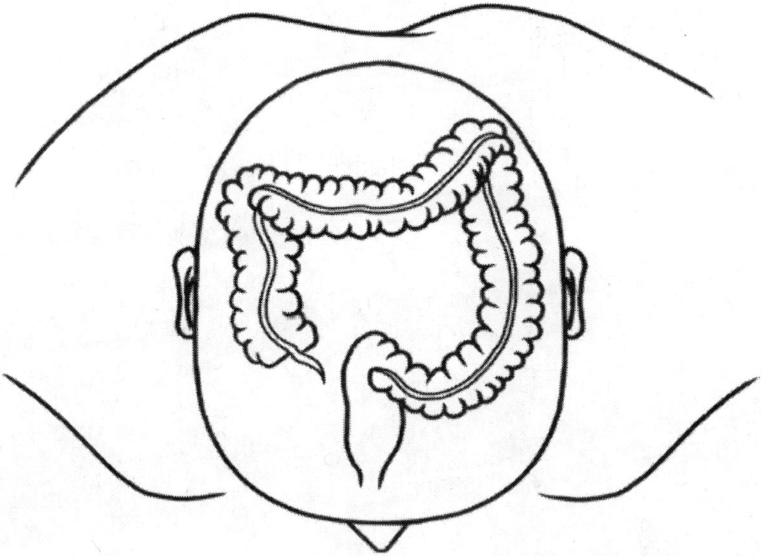

Figure 1.15 The contour of the top of the head is related to the large intestine

2

The head

Functional anatomy of the ki in the head

The head is related to our entire life, manifesting through pains our difficulties with a happening located in our history or even an early concern with something in our future.

Past: The posterior part of the head up to the base of the cranium corresponds to our past. Pains in this region indicate emotional problems related to the person's past (see Figure 2.1).

Present: Tracing an imaginary line from one ear to the other, passing through the top of the head, in a range of about nine centimeters, we identify the area corresponding to problems related to the present.

Future: Tracing another imaginary line from one temple to the other, passing over the head up to the forehead, we find the area corresponding to problems in the future. People with pains in this region are usually anxious and can manifest gastric problems and nervous ulcers.

Therefore, when the person has pain in a part of the head, we can related it, according to its loca

tion, to an occurrence in the past, a difficulty faced in the present or a concern with something in the future (see Figure 2.1).

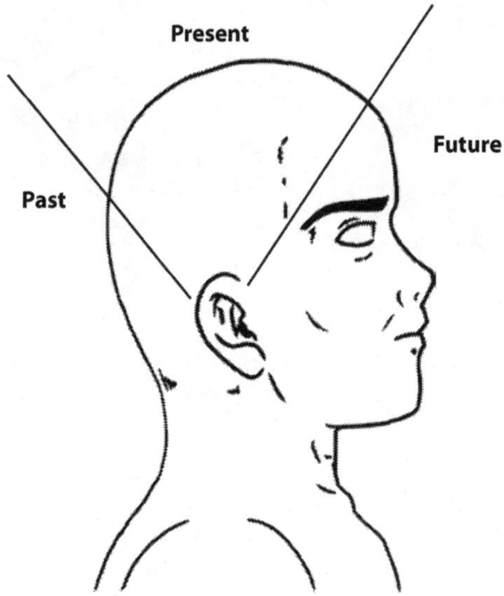

Figure 2.1 The time relations in the head

The entire right hemisphere corresponds to the yang part: practical, analytical, masculine; while the left hemisphere is related to the *yin* part: creative, emotional, feminine.

The right part of the head also corresponds to the liver, kidney and large intestine. While the left part corresponds to the stomach, spleen, pancreas and lungs.

The top of the head

In the head, we find several points to stimulate the nervous system, the internal organs and sight. Treatment in the head should be done gently, always aiming at reducing tension of the neck, which makes the head "heavy".

The type of thinking of the person influences the tension of the neck's musculature. When the head is "heavy", it is because the ki is stagnant. The person has negative thoughts and feels anguished. Likewise, when the thoughts are freer, calm, constructive, positive, the musculature of the neck relaxes, the head becomes lighter and this favors a deeper breathing.

One can perceive this by inducing the person to think of a tranquil beach, with fresh air. We then see that the head changes its weight.

Hya kue: the point of a thousand diseases

Right in the center of the head, we find a tsubo (vital, energy point) of great importance, known by the Japanese as hya kue, the VG20, a point that belongs to the meridian of the governing vessel. It is also called the "point of a thousand diseases" or "point of a hundred meetings", since it is used to treat several types of imbalances (see Figure 2.2). We resort to this point in cases of stress, insomnia, anxiety, depression, addictions (smoking and alcohol), hemorrhoids and inflammations.

Points related to the ovaries

On the top of the head, there are also points to treat the ovaries. The points beside the hya kue (right and left) represent each one of the ovaries respectively (see Figure 2.2).

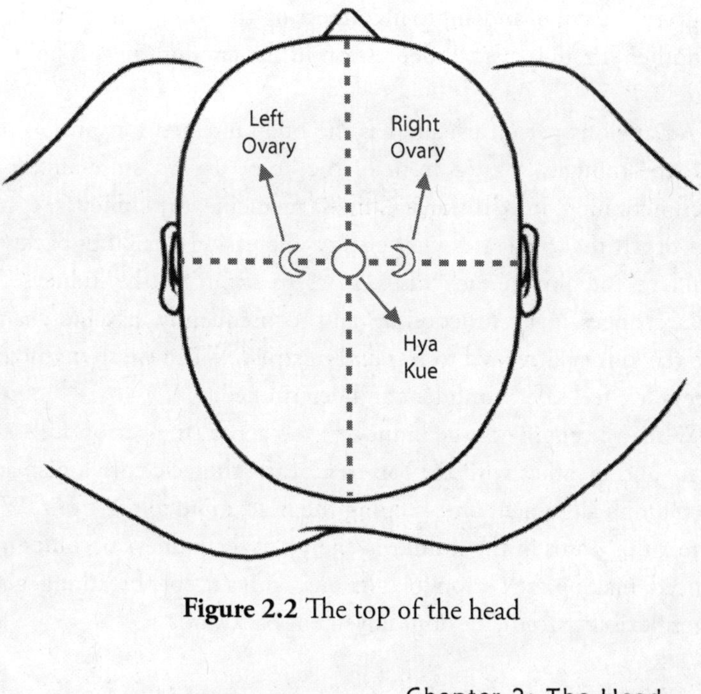

Figure 2.2 The top of the head

Diagnosis

With the person lying down with the abdomen facing up, with the knees flexed and the feet together, in the butterfly position, check which knee is high, indicating that the pelvis is bent to this side. This indicates that the ovary on the same side is altered. The bent pelvis also interferes in the proper functioning of the ovaries.

Treatment

In this case, we must stimulate the point of the ovary that will, in general, be painful or more sensitive to touch (see Figure 2.2). This treatment is also indicates in cases of premenstrual stress (PMS) and problems in the menstrual cycle. it is also effective in cases of polyps in the ovaries.

Posterior part of the head

In the posterior part of the head, we find two very effective points for the kidneys. Each point represents a kidney and is located in the intersection of two lines: one coming from the eye, passing over the head and reaching up to the nape, and another connecting the top of an ear to the top of another. There is a small depression in the cranium in this point (see Figure 2.3).

An anxious person usually has the body inclined forward, as if the head, the thought, was in front of the body. This posture affects kidneys functioning. In traditional Chinese medicine, the kidney is regarded as an organ that generates vital energy. Increasing flexibility backwards should be the aim in such cases, so as to stimulate the kidneys. This causes changes in its functioning and, consequently, psychic changes, since the kidney is related to fear and mistrust. When we strengthen our kidneys, we feel safer, confident and determined.

When the energy of the kidneys is too active, the person feels more anxiety and breathes with the top part of the thoracic cavity, displacing the column's alignment and keeping the head more to the front. When we treat this point in the head, the energy of the kidneys becomes more balanced, making the person less anxious, with a deeper breathing, giving greater flexibility to the flexion movement backwards.

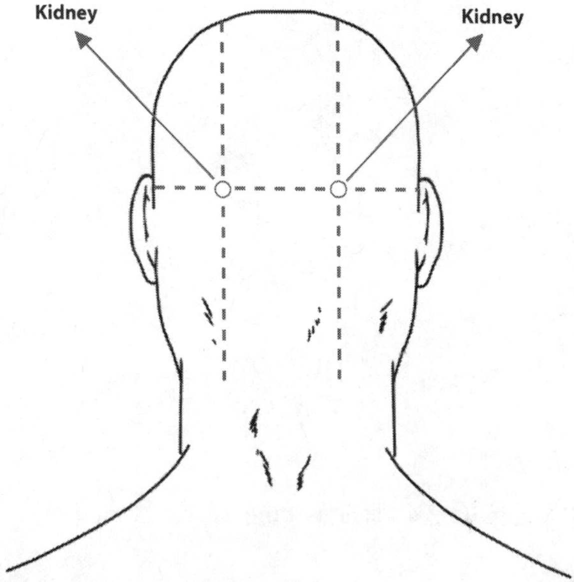

Figure 2.3 Points related to the kidneys in the head

Diagnosis

Standing, the person must flex the body as much as possible backwards and check how far he/she can see and the state of his/her posterior flexibility (see Figure 2.4). He/she must notice if he/she feels difficulty on performing this movement.

Treatment

With the person lying down in ventral decubitus, that is, with the stomach facing down, stimulate at least 20 times the points of the kidney in the posterior part of the head (see Figure 2.3).

On repeating the flexion movement backwards, the person will notice a greater flexibility and ease in practicing this movement. Stimulation in these points causes a relaxation in the posterior musculature of the back and region of the kidneys, in addition to also treating the energy of these organs. On stimulating this point, breathing becomes deeper.

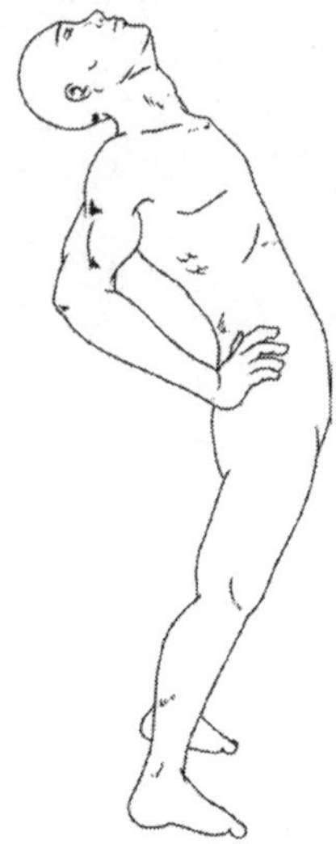

Figure 2.4 Flexion of the body backwards

Kidneys and ears

In the ears we finds points of the whole body, but they are specifically related to the kidneys. Changes in color and sensitivity of the ears, that is, when they are redder or more sensitive, or even painful, indicate a contracted kidney, with much jitsu energy, which can indicate a tendency to develop gallstones.

We can treat the kidneys through the ears. On massaging them, we are stimulating the kidneys.

Diagnosis

With the person lying down in the locust pose, as shown in Figure 2.5, note the height of each leg in relation to the floor. It is common for the legs to have different heights, also indicating a difference in the condition of each kidney.

Treatment

Rub each ear with the hands, at least 100 times. Finally, ask the person to do the locust pose again and check if the legs are freer to rise. Usually, this mere rubbing of the ears is able to balance the heights of the legs.

Another way of diagnosing the functioning of the kidney is through the urine. When the urine comes out like a strong jet, this indicates good renal functioning. Otherwise, when the urine comes out with a disperse and weak jet, this indicates malfunctioning of the kidney. In such cases, we can stimulate the kidneys through the points mentioned above and by rubbing the years.

Base of the cranium

The lower median part of the head, where the center of the base of the cranium is located, is related to the genital organs. It is specially indicated for the treatment of premenstrual stress symptoms, menstrual cramps and for the treatment of prostate.

The sides of the base of the cranium are related to the left and right legs respectively (see Figure 2.6).

Diagnosis

The person must stretch a leg and flex the other, inclining the body to the side, in the yoga janu sir-sasana pose (see Figure 2.7). Identify the less flexible side of the torso, the side with the most difficulty to incliner the body along the leg.

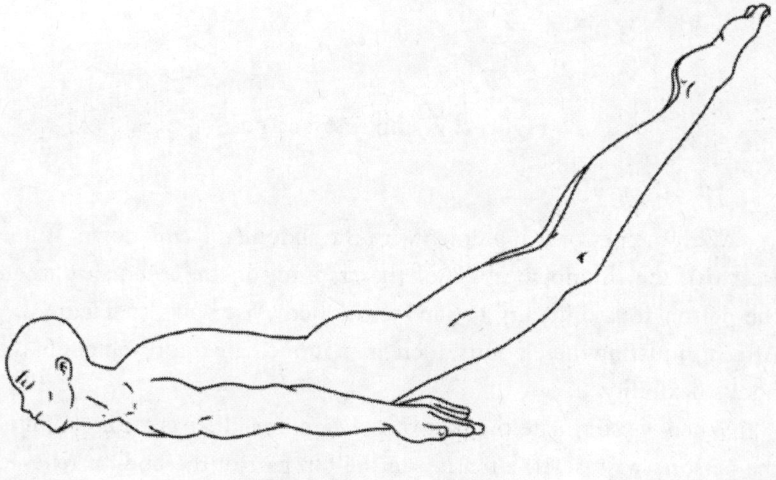

Figure 2.5 Locust Pose

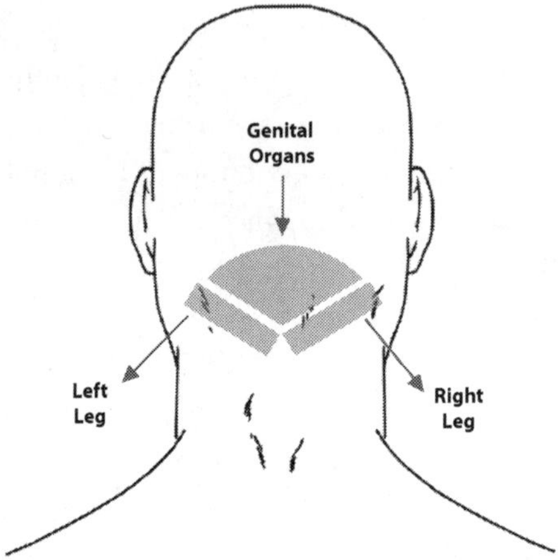

Figure 2.6 Relationships of the base of the cranium

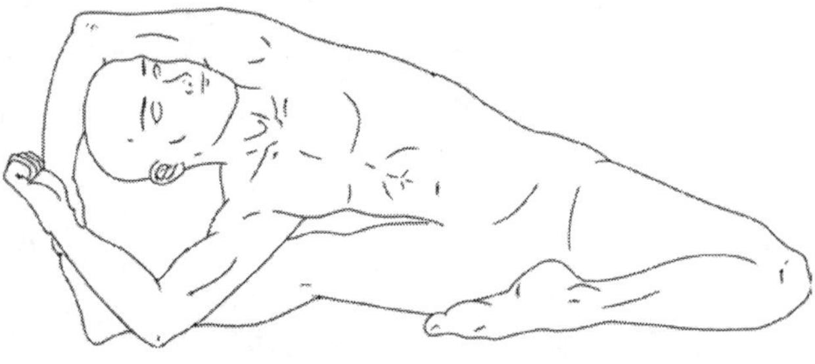

Figure 2.7 Janu sirsasana pose

Treatment

With the person lying down with the abdomen facing down, stimulate with the thumb the base of the cranium on the same side where the person feels difficulty to incline the body, as shown in Figure 2.6. After stimulating these points, there is an immediate improvement in the body's flexibility.

When we stimulate the base of the cranium, there is a correction in the person's posture. The tension in the top part of the body is relieved and the base, in the lumbar region and legs, is strengthened.

Gert's recovery

Testimony by Fernando Montoto

In Japan, in the 80s, I had the opportunity of witnessing the treatment of a student called Gert. Gert was Belgian and had gone to live in the dojo, in Mishima, to be treated by Oki sensei. He had a lot of difficulty to move, used crutches and showed a generalized weakness of the legs. His musculature was very flaccid and he staggered on trying to walk.

Oki sensei treated him through the points in the lower part of the cranium, which are specific points for strengthening of the legs. Gert lived in the dojo for six months and was always treated by Oki sensei with emphasis on the pressure of these points at the base of the cranium. At the end of three months, Gert stopped using the crutches and was already able to walk.

Oki sensei would say to Gert that he had this difficulty to walk due to the overprotection of his parents. His legs became very weak, as if he was unable to walk with them. After six months of living in the dojo, Gert returned to his country. I took him to the train station. While I waited for him in the car, he said goodbye to the people, took two bags and came running toward the car.

The image of Gert running with his bags toward me was recorded for ever in my memory.

The sight of Takamuki

Testimony by Fernando Montoto and Paula Guimarães

It was the spring of 1986 when Takamuki arrived in the dojo in Mishima, Japan. Coming from Hokkaido, he used eyeglasses with 6 degrees of myopia. He had a lot of difficulty to see and drive his Datsun, a car he brought from his native city. He spoke English well and soon became friends with the gaijin group, we the foreigners.

During his stay at the dojo, he would sit every morning stimulating certain points of his face, which we will describe in this chapter (see Figures 2.8 and 2.9). Together with this, he practiced a series of correctional exercises that aimed at stretching and relaxing the musculature of the shoulders and upper part of his body. According to oriental medicine, the tension and hardening of the shoulder musculature impairs the muscles of sight, just as sight is related to the liver and gallbladder.

Takamuki practiced exercises, pressed the points and also cared for his liver through an integral and balanced diet we ate in the dojo.

After six months of practice, he passed a test in the driving school, this time without eyeglasses. Not only had his sight improved, but his self-confidence as well, since the exercises indicated for the sight are connected to the upper part of the body and thoracic cavity. After one year of training and treatment, his vision improved greatly and he no longer used eyeglasses. Takamuki also changed his vision of the world and future, returning to Hokkaido with many ideas to be developed. Twenty-two years later, in the spring of 2008, we came across Takamuki again in Japan. He had gray hair, the same broad smile and he was without eyeglasses.

Points for sight

The points to follow are located in the face and head, are indicated for treatment of sight problems, like myopia, hypermetropia, tired sight and others (see Figures 2.8 and 2.9). They can also be used to rest the eyes, taking some intervals after a long period at the computer, sewing, reading, driving an automobile in a highway, in short, it is advisable to press them during any activity that requires more effort from the sight.

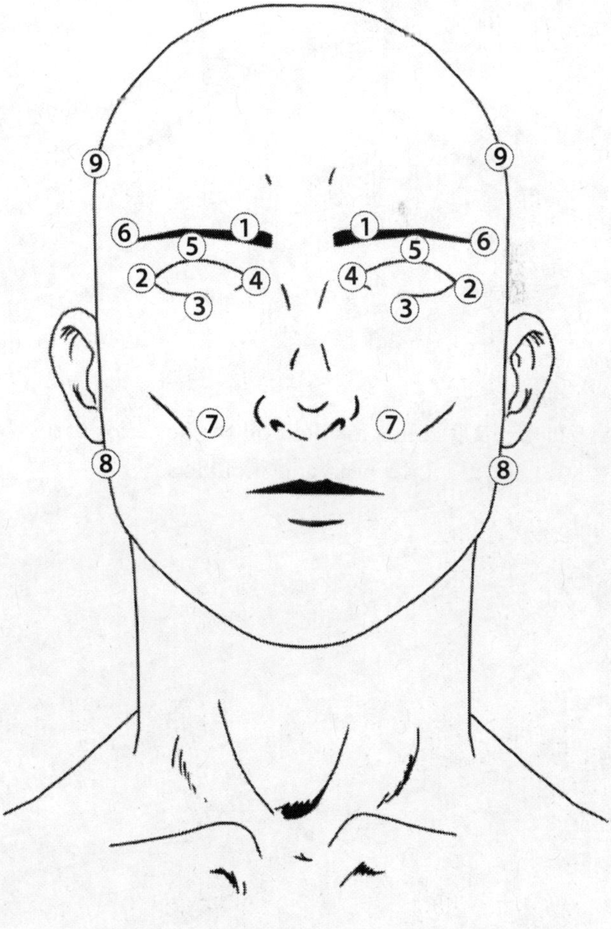

Figure 2.8 Points for sight on the face

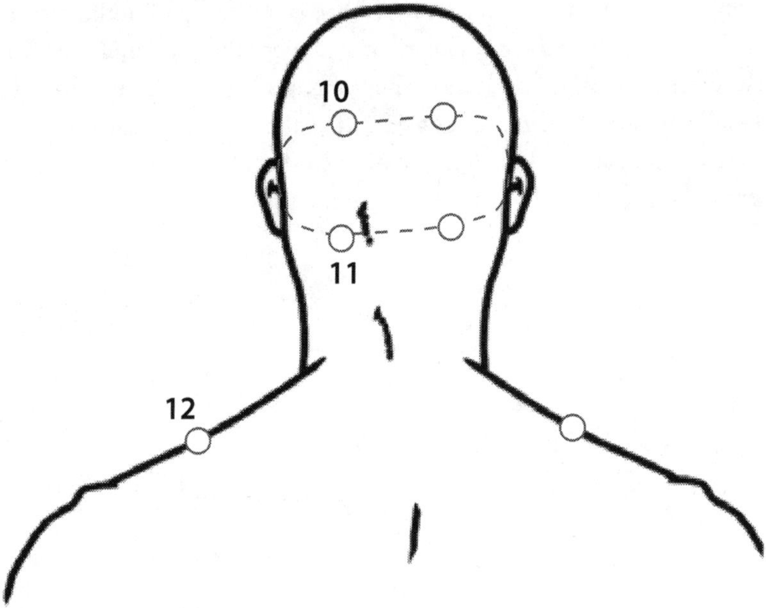

Figure 2.9 Points for sight on the posterior part of the head and shoulders

Each point of the sight must be pressed with the flesh of the thumb and/or middle finger at least 20 times. These points must be treated daily:

1. Look for a fissure or depression in the frontal bone, one centimeter from the beginning of the eyelash, in the upper part of the eye cavity;
2. In the outer lateral part of the eye, as well as in the outer corner of the eye cavity;
3. In the center of the lower part of the eye where there is a small depression or fissure in the bone;
4. In the upper part of the nose, in the point where the forehead meets the nose;
5. In the center of the upper part of the eye, where there is also a depression in the bone;
6. At the end of the eyelash;
7. Beside the nostrils, press the cheek of the face upwards;
8. In the cavity between the lower jaw and the sternocleidomastoid muscle, in the neck, right below the ear;
9. In the region of the temples, where the scalp beings;
10. If we trace an imaginary line from the eye up to the nape and another line linking the center of one ear to the other, the points of the kidneys are found in the intersection of the lines, as we have already seen in the chapter on the head. This is also a point for sight;
11. On the posterior side of the base of the cranium there is point number 20 of the *meridian* of the gallbladder;
12. In the upper part of the trapezius, where there is point 21 of the *meridian* of the gallbladder.

3

THE FEET

The feet have the capacity to relax our entire posture, more specifically our spinal column. In this chapter, we will discuss the points located on the sole of the feet, related to each one of the vertebrae of the spine, as shown in Figure 3.1.

An interesting way of diagnosing the posture is through the sole of the shoes. If we note the sole of the shoes, in some cases, we see that they are more worn out on one side than on the other. When the sole of the shoe is worn out in the external lateral part, this indicates a certain tension in the cervical region and in the shoulders. While if the sole of the shoe is more worn out in the inner side of the feet, this indicates certain tension in the lumbar region.

Another way of diagnosing is by investigating where the person has callousness or painful parts in the feet. Relate the area with callousness or pain with the points of Figure 3.1. The callous place indicates a problem in the corresponding vertebra. For example, a person with a callousness in the plantar part of the foot, near the toes, can have a cyphosis in the top

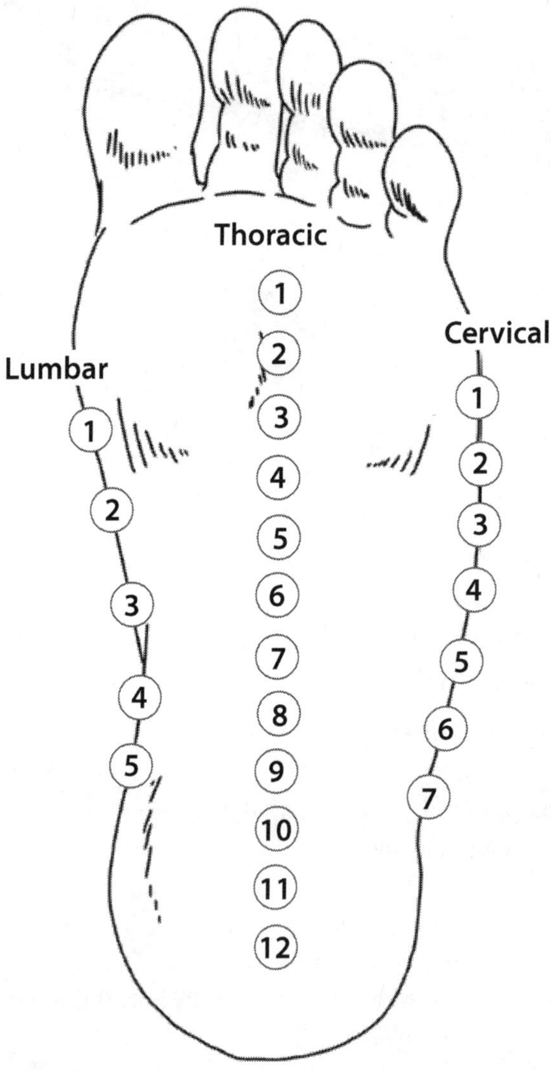

Figure 3.1 Points for the spinal column in the sole of the foot

part of the thoracic cavity or pains in the musculature of this region.

A good massage in the feet will give a feeling of relief in the physical posture, relaxing the body and mind, stimulating the parasympathetic nervous system and providing a deep sleep.

In the case of the hands and feet, there is in *kanrenbui* a series of practices aimed at improving the flexibility and symmetry of the physical body, thus giving the human being an equilibrium. In this chapter, we will show some of these practices related to the feet.

It is important to note that these stimuli can be practiced in the feet without the exercise that accompanies it. In fact, the exercise aims at showing how the stimulus in the point immediately changes the movement related to the vertebra to be treated. However, we can also use this map of the feet from *kanrenbui* to treat any disorder, pain or tension in the spine. In our more than 25 years of clinical experience, we were able to notice that the best way to treat pains and problems in the spine is by following this map of the feet from *kanrenbui.*

Relation of the vertebrae with the feet
Lumbar region

Lumbar 1 and 5

People who have difficulty to stretch the spine forward have complications in lumbar vertebrae 1 and 5 (L1 & L5), which in turn are related to the brain. Stimulus of the points related to these two vertebrae, located in the region of the arch of the foot increases flexibility. The points must be pressed about 30 times.

Lumbar vertebrae L1 & L5 are related to movement of the spine of flexion forward and backward. They are also related to the mind. People with very stiff minds have great difficulty to flex the body back and forward. They have a breathing more located in the top part of the thorax and use only a small part of their lung capacity. A limited breathing causes the thinking to also be limited, with difficulty to adapt to new situations, becoming a person with little adaptability. The tendency is for these people to become stiff in their thinking also, cultivating fixed ideas, which can cause certain suffering in them, since life is ever changing. Increased flexibility in the spine makes the nervous system more balanced and the mind more flexible.

Treatment for lumbar 1 and 5

While standing, check up to where the person can flex the body forward, with the knees stretched, as shown in Figure 3.3.

With the person lying down with the abdomen facing down, press the point in the foot related to lumbar 1 and 5 (see Figure 3.2).

Check the first position of the flexion movement of the spine forward again. The person will feel more ease in flexing.

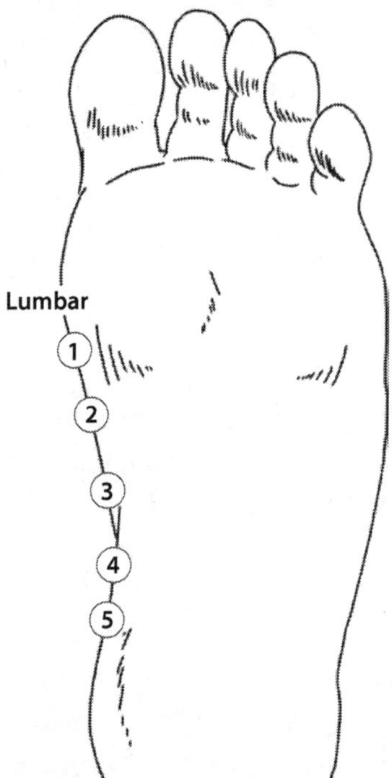

Figure 3.2 Points related to the lumbar vertebrae in the foot

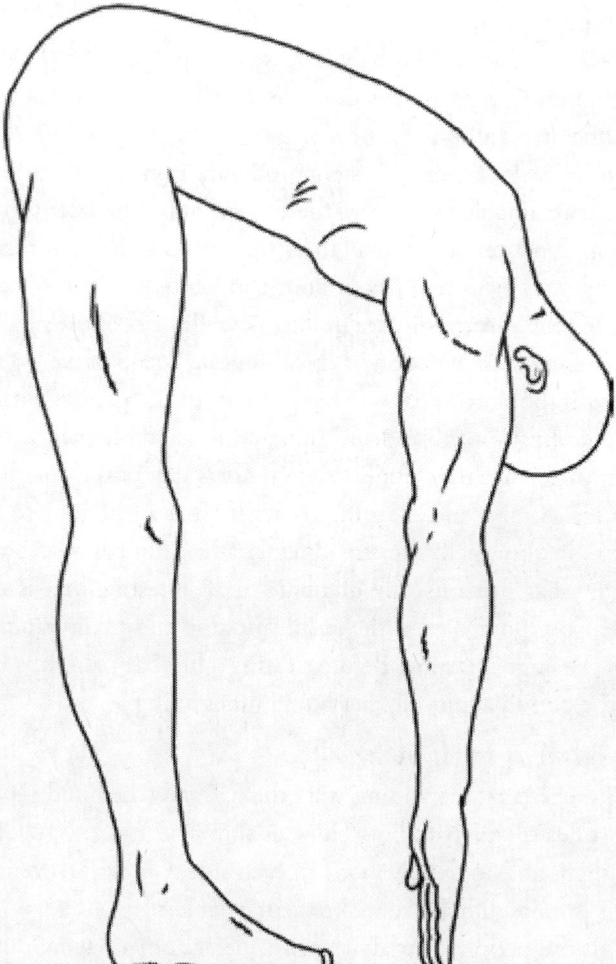

Figure 3.3 Flexion of the body forward

Lumbar 2

Lumbar vertebra 2 (L2) is related to the lateral movement of the spinal column. When the person has difficulty to flex the body to the sides, we must treat the points of L2 in both feet.

L2 is also related to digestion and absorption of foods and the intestines. We can use this point

of L2 in the arch of both feet to also treat people with poor digestion. We also use this point to treat people with anemia or osteoporosis, who have difficulty to absorb the iron or calcium and magnesium respectively. Many people with anemia or osteoporosis take iron or calcium and magnesium, but are unable to improve these symptoms. This occurs because the absorbing function of the small intestine is not balanced. It may be dirty, retaining in its walls residues of flour and white rice or processed foods, preventing the absorption area in the microvilosities of the small intestine from fulfilling their function of absorbing the nutrients we ingest. In this case, it is important to have a change in diet. The person must begin to eat whole cereals, like bread and rice, and flaxseed blended with fruits in the morning, since these foods contain fibers that pass through the small intestine sweeping and cleaning its walls. It is important to note that problems in the small intestine directly affect lumbar vertebra number 2. The lumbar pains usually originate in an intestine that is dirty with residues from poor diet in the small intestine and toxins from previous feces in the large intestine. Before treating a lumbar pain, it is important to ask the person about his/ her bowel functioning.

Treatment for lumbar 2

With the person standing with the legs stretched and separate, he/ she must flex the body to both sides, as shown in Figure 3.4. Check how far he/ she is able to flex the body to each side. Check if there is a side to which it is more difficult to make the movement.

With the person lying down with the abdomen facing down, press the points related to lumbar 2 in both feet (see Figure 3.2), giving more emphasis to that which is more painful or to the foot opposite the less flexible side of the body.

After pressing 20 times on breathing out, check the first position again with lateral flexion of the body. You will notice the increase in flexibility and greater ease of lateral movement, especially to the side that had greater difficulty.

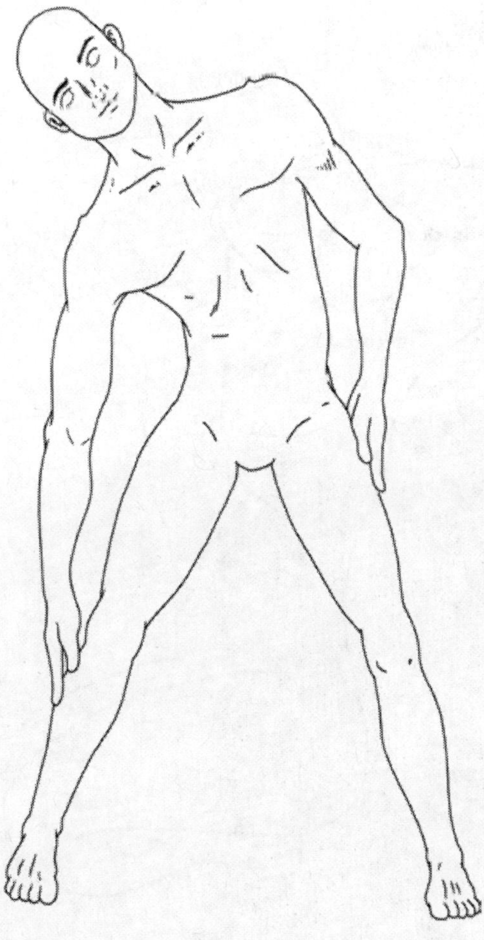

Figure 3.4 Lateral flexion of the body

Lumbar 3

Lumbar vertebra 3 (L3) is related to the bending movement of the body to both sides.

People with difficulty to bend the body, regardless of the side, have a stiffness in lumbar vertebra number 3.

L3 is also associated with the kidneys and knees. People with pains in the knees have much difficulty in making a bending movement of the body.

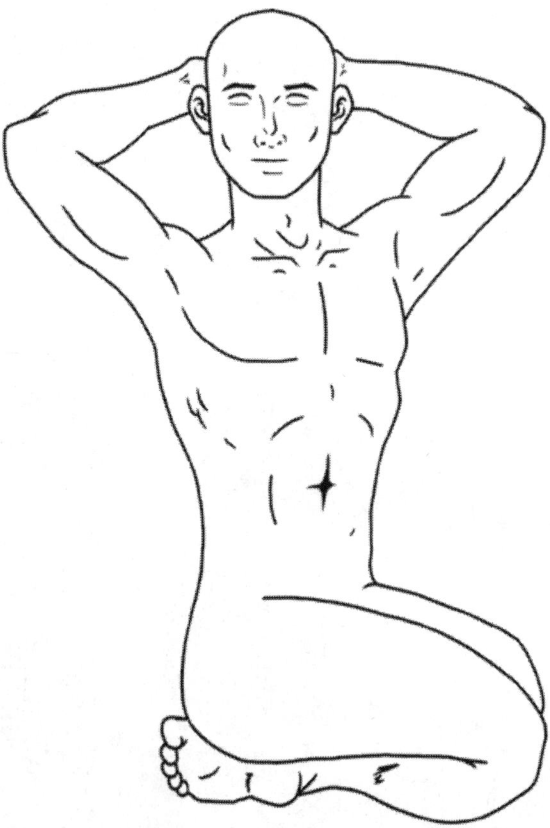

Figure 3.5 Bending of the body

When the kidney is too overburdened, the person becomes anxious, the body is projected forward, making it difficult to perform the bending movement. Therefore, we can use this point in the feet to treat the condition of the kidneys.

Lumbar vertebra number 3 is located at the height of the navel. When the musculature beside L3 is too high (yang) on one side than another (yin), we must press the center of the arch of the foot corresponding to the side where the musculature is low, the yin side. We will thus cause a balance in the lumbar musculature, thus improving the hip's position.

Treatment for lumbar 3

Sitting in *seiza*, with the hands intertwined behind the head, the person must bend the body to one side and to the other, trying to see the farthest point possible with the bending movement (see Figure 3.5).

With the person lying down with the abdomen facing down, the therapist must press, in the foot, the point related to lumbar 3. It must be located in the center of the arch line of the feet (see Figure 3.2). Both feet must be pressed, however, giving greater attention to the one with more pain.

Check the first position again. The person will feel more ease in performing the bending movement.

When the musculature of one side of the lumbar differs from that of the other, this interferes in the pelvis' rotation. For example, when the musculature of the right side is tense and that of the left side is relaxed, we must work, in this case, all the arch of the foot from the same side of the relaxed musculature, that is, the arch of the left foot. With the treatment in the foot, the musculature that is more relaxed or low will be raised. This will change the aspect of the musculature in the lumbar region, thus correcting the hip's position.

Lumbar 4

Lumbar 4 (L4) is related to movement of opening the legs and pelvis. People with stagnant energy or stiffness in lumbar 4 have difficulty to sit on the floor, especially if they must sit with the legs open or folded in the lotus position.

Lumbar 4 is also related to the sexual organs and with the entire pelvic region. When the person has menstrual problems, like menstrual cramps, PMS, impotence or stiffness, we must use this point in both feet. The movement of opening and closing the pelvis is related to the genital organs.

Treatment for lumbar 4

With the person sitting on the floor with the legs open, check up to where he/she can open the legs, marking this opening, as shown in Figure 3.6.

With the person lying down with the tummy facing down, the therapist must press the point in the arch of the foot related to lumbar 4, in both feet, pressing the foot in which the more sensitive point is located for a longer time (see Figure 3.2).

Ask the person to sit again and check the opening of the legs. The movement of opening the legs will be better and he/she will be able to open them wider.

People who sit with difficulty in the lotus position will feel greater ease to make the pose if the points of lumbar 4 are worked.

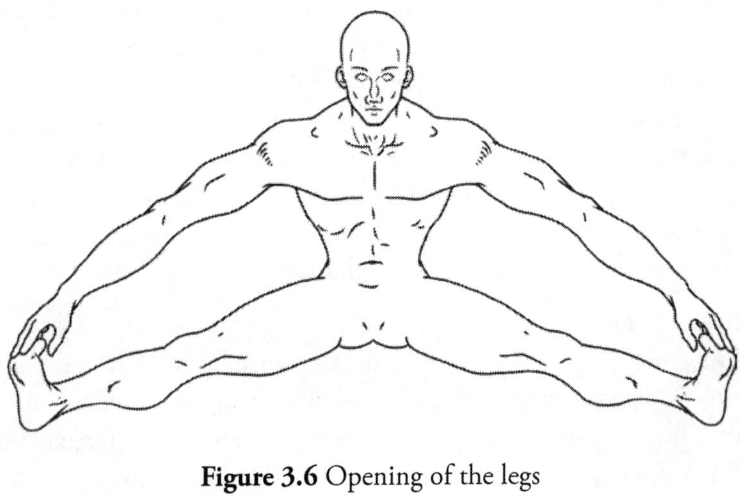

Figure 3.6 Opening of the legs

Thoracic or dorsal region

The entire region of the thoracic vertebrae has a relation with the median line of the foot. Changes in the paravertebral musculature and some pains in the thoracic region can be treated in the sole of the foot, in the area corresponding to the vertebra or affected region, as shown in Figure 3.7.

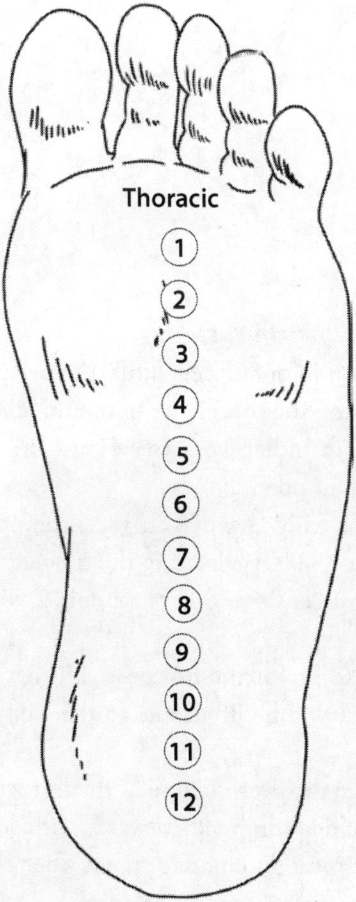

Figura 3.7 Area corresponding to the vertebra or affected region

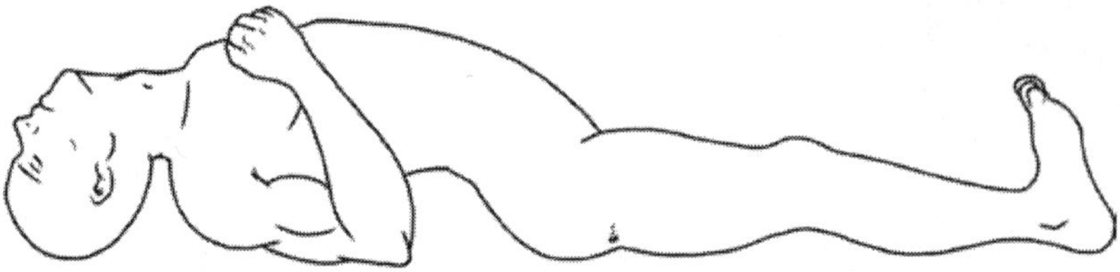

Figure 3.8 Fish pose

Treatment for the thoracic region:

While lying down in dorsal decubitus, the person must lift the thoracic cavity, supporting the top of the head and elbows on the ground: this is the fish pose, in Indian yoga (see Figure 3.8). We can check the chest's expansion in this pose.

With the person lying down with the abdomen facing down, we must press the line in the feet related to the thoracic cavity, paying more attention to the most sensitive points or points with pain (see Figure 3.7).

Ask the person to repeat the fish pose. His/her thoracic cavity will expand and the chest will be lifted due to the stimulus in the thoracic vertebrae.

We must massage the thoracic line in the feet whenever the person's chest is closed, shoulders dropped forward, with lung problems or in depressive states. We must also massage them when there is a problem in the thoracic region of the spine, such as a scoliosis, cyphosis or muscular tension, very common between the scapulae and spinal column.

Cervical region

The outer lateral parts of the foot are related to the cervix. People who wear out the sole of the shoe in this area indicate a very tense posture in the shoulder and neck. Cervical vertebrae 1 to 7 have their points related in the side, starting from the little toe up to the heel (see Figure 3.9).

Treatment for the cervical region

While standing or sitting, the person must bend the neck to the right and left in order to know which side is more difficult, according to Figure 3.10.

With the person lying down with the abdomen facing down, work the outer side of the foot opposite the more difficult side, where there are the points related to the cervical vertebrae, looking for

the more sensitive and painful points and stimulating them with the thumb approximately 30 times (see Figure 3.9).

With the person standing or sitting, check the movement of bending the neck again. Check how more flexible it is.

This stimulation in the points of the cervix located in the feet must be applied when there is much tension in the cervical region, stiff neck, protrusion or disk hernia in the cervical vertebrae. One must also massage these points a lot in people who spend many hours in front of the computer and people with sight problems who tend to have a tenser cervical region.

The toes and lumbar vertebrae

The toes are related with each one of the lumbar vertebrae. From the biggest to the smallest, they are connected to lumbar 1 to 5 respectively.

Lumbar 1 and 5

As we have already seen, on studying the relation of the lumbar vertebrae in the feet, lumbar L1 and L5 are related to the anterior and posterior flexion movement, that is, bending the body forward and backward.

In people with difficulty to bend the spine forward, work, in each foot, the big toe or hallux and the small toe, connected to lumbar 1 and

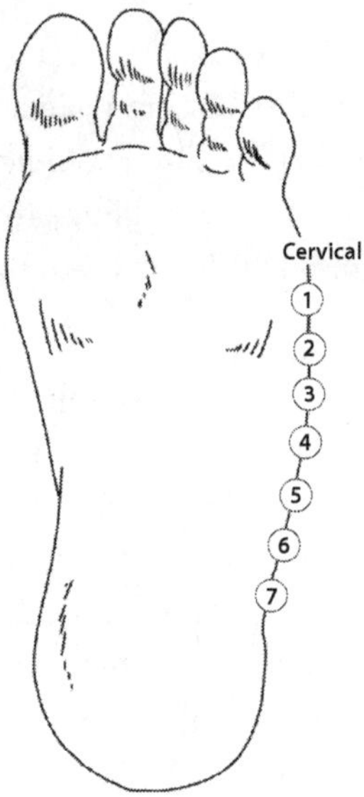

Figura 3.9 Area corresponding

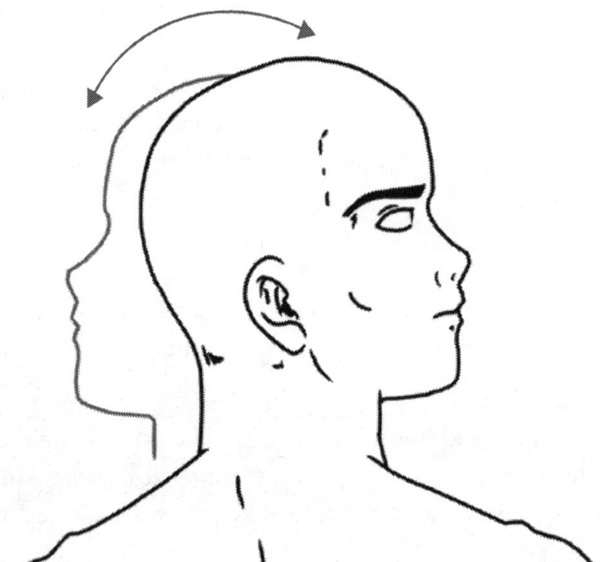

Figure 3.10 Bending of the cervix

5 (see Figure 3.11) respectively, with circular movements (20 times in both directions). Bend to both sides and pull the toes strongly. This will increase flexibility of the spine forward and backward.

Lumbar 2

In people with difficulty to flex the spine to the right and left, we must work the second toe of each foot, related to L2 (see Figure 3.11). If the person has difficulty to flex the body to the right, work the second toe of the left foot more than the right. If there is difficulty to flex the body to the left, work more on the second toe of the right foot. After stimulating the toes, check if there was increase in flexibility.

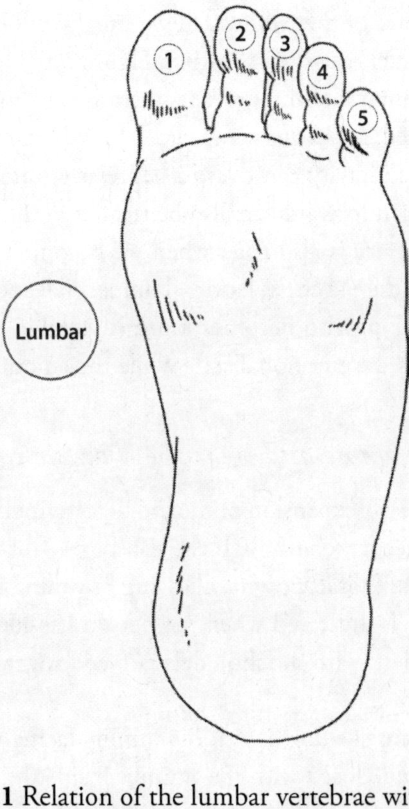

Figure 3.11 Relation of the lumbar vertebrae with the toes

Lumbar 3

People with difficulty to make the bending movement of the spine to the right or left side have problems or merely a stiffness or stagnant energy in lumbar number 3. Work the third finger with circular movements (see Figure 3.11), bending and stretching.

Lumbar 4

The fourth toe is related to lumbar 4 (see Figure 3.11), connected to the movement of opening the legs. The various stimuli in the fourth toe of both feet will relax the legs, providing greater flexibility and ease in opening them.

The back of the foot and thoracic cavity

The anterior surface of the feet, which we usually call back of the foot, is related to the thoracic cavity, as shown in Figure 3.12. Tension in the musculature of the thoracic cavity prevents it from expanding. Thus, breathing is compromised, appearing symptomatically as a superficial breathing. The closed thoracic cavity can cause a depressive state. The closed chest and shoulders fallen forward can also be treated in the anterior region of the feet. The contrary is also true: when we become depressed, we have the tendency to close the chest, let the shoulders fall and contract the thoracic cavity. Our lung also becomes more vulnerable to infirmities. The posture influences the emotional state while the emotion state influences the posture.

Exercise to diagnose and treat the thoracic cavity: fish pose

We can check the expansion of the thoracic cavity through breathing, which becomes deeper, or through the fish pose. This will stimulate the musculature of the thoracic cavity, allowing breathing to flow deeper.

The fish pose is indicated when the person has superficial breathing and contracted chest, with the shoulders curved forward, since it expands the thoracic cavity.

The person must lie down with the tummy facing up, with the arms flexed and the hand closed with the thumbs inside the fingers. With the elbows supported on the floor, push only the thorax up, also supporting the top of the head on the floor. The hip must remain on the floor, with the legs stretched and the Achilles tendon stretched (see Figure 3.13).

With the hand thrust into the gap between the floor and thoracic vertebrae, measure the space there; check how far the thorax is able to lift from the floor.

This asana alone, which is a pose from yoga, is an exercise for opening and expansion of the thoracic cavity. However, if we press the points of kanrenbui related to the thoracic cavity on the back of the foot, the expansion effect will be surprisingly greater.

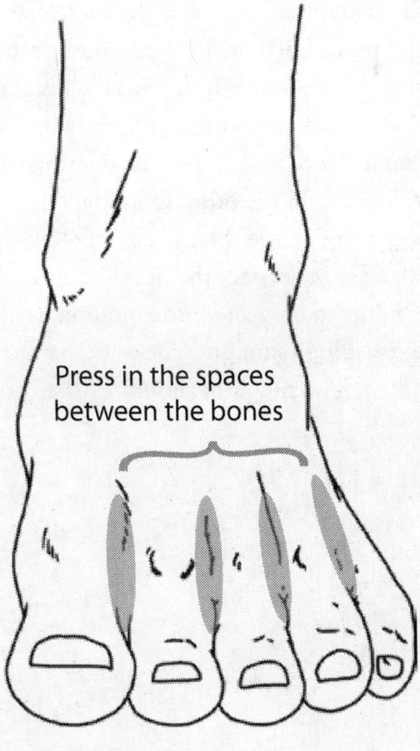

Figure 3.12 Points related to the thoracic cavity on the back of the foot

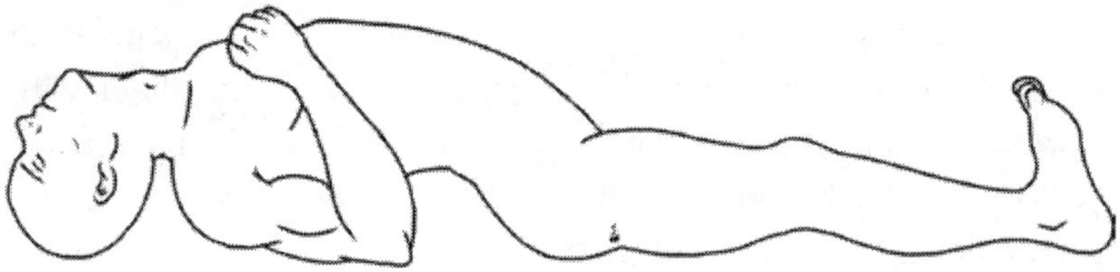

Figure 3.13 Fish pose

Treatment for the thoracic cavity

On the back of the foot, between the metatarsus (the bones of the feet that form the toes), find the most painful or sensitive point in each valley, that is, in each line between the metatarsus (see Figure 3.12), and press it at least 20 times on breathing out.

Repeat the same procedure in all four lines between the bones. Perform the same treatment in the other foot.

In Japan, we learned to use the analogy of the valleys and mountains in the whole body. The valleys are the depressions in the body, where we usually find the points to be treated; the mountains are the bones.

Practice the fish pose again and check how much the thoracic cavity expanded and by how much flexibility of the thoracic vertebrae increased.

4

The legs

In the legs, we find many points related to the internal organs. Swelling, poor circulation or varices in the legs indicate malfunctioning of the internal organs, since, when these are expanded, blood circulation in the legs becomes deficient and venous return of the blood becomes difficult. The tendency is for the feet to become cold in such cases.

The cause of this problem is the fallen or flaccid organs. Usually, people with this characteristic have a very *kyo* abdomen (empty) in the upper part and *jitsu* (full) in the lower part. When the organs from the lower part are full, stiff, fallen, blood circulation in the legs becomes difficult. On pressing the organs from the lower part, we can notice the change in the arteries, that is, a strong pulsation in the abdomen. This pulsation in the abdominal region is a symptom of stomach prolapse or, as we usually call it, fallen organs.

Points related to the pelvis and sexual organs

There is a relation between the sexual organs and the pelvis with the inner part of the legs. Placing the hand in the pubic region, the little finger indicates a very effective point to treat genital problems (see Figure 4.1). In the case of women, this point is used to treat inflammations or polyps in the ovaries and problems in the uterus; in men, it is used for the prostate and sexual organs.

The movement of opening the legs and pelvis is related to the sexual organs. When the person's pelvis is too closed and there is no flexibility in opening the legs, this shows an imbalance in the sexual organs.

Diagnosis

By pressing the low tummy, the low and mid region of the abdomen, a little above the pubis, with the middle fingers of both hands, check which side is tenser. Usually, the hipbone on this side is higher. In this region, we diagnose the ovaries and uterus through touch. Also note the position of the iliac crests, identifying which is higher.

Treatment

Press the point in Figure 4.1 approximately 30 times in the inner part of the tight, revealed by the little finger. The pressure can be exerted with the thumb or with the palm of the hand.

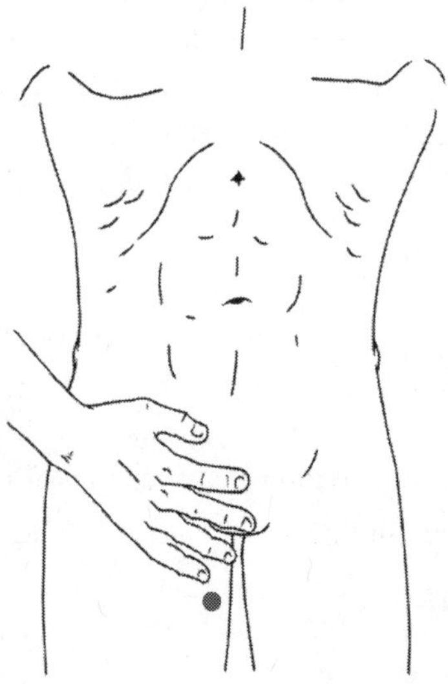

Figure 4.1 Points related to the pelvis and sexual organs

Points for treatment of internal organs

Intestines

There is a relation between the large intestine and inner part of the legs, a little above the knees. In this region, there are some very efficient points for treatment of pains in the low region of the abdomen, very near the iliac crests, as shown in figure 4.2.

Diagnosis

Press with the middle fingers of both hands the area located between the navel and iliac crest, starting from the lower part of the abdomen, finding the stiffest or painful points from one side to the other.

Treatment

Look for the related point in the inner part of the leg, from the same side where there is pain in the abdomen, a little above the knee (see Figure 4.2). This point will be more sensitive and with pain. Stimulate it 20 times with the thumb or palm of the hand. Next, check if the stiffness or pain in the low lateral region of the abdomen is more reduced.

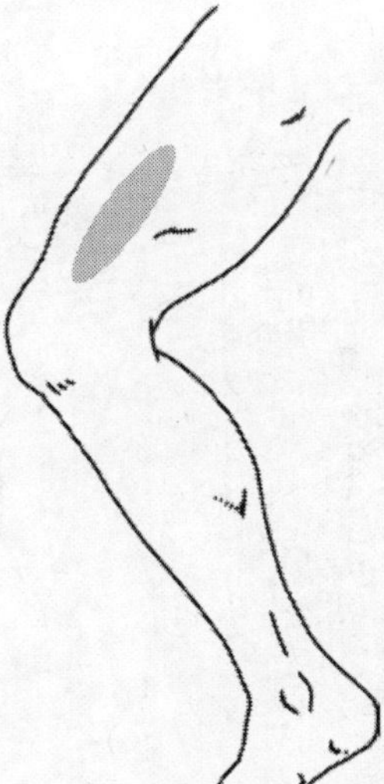

Figure 4.2 Part related to the large intestine

Liver

In the outer part of the leg, there is an important point for treatment of the liver. It is recommended in cases in which this organ has too much *jitsu, yang,* increased in size, when people consume too much alcohol or fried food. People with constipation always have a *jitsu* condition in the liver. As already mentioned previously, constipation causes the organism to absorb a great amount of toxins, which will later be filtered by the liver, overburdening this organ. The feelings of anger, frustration, extreme self-criticism or a deep demand from oneself affect the liver, leaving it more yang.

Diagnosis

With the person lying down with the tummy facing up, press the top part of the abdomen below the ribs from the right side, where there is the liver and gallbladder, as shown in Figure 4.3. This pressure must be made with the middle fingers of both hands together. Press three points from the center outwards of the abdomen, noting if there is a more painful or stiff point, indicating a poor condition of the liver.

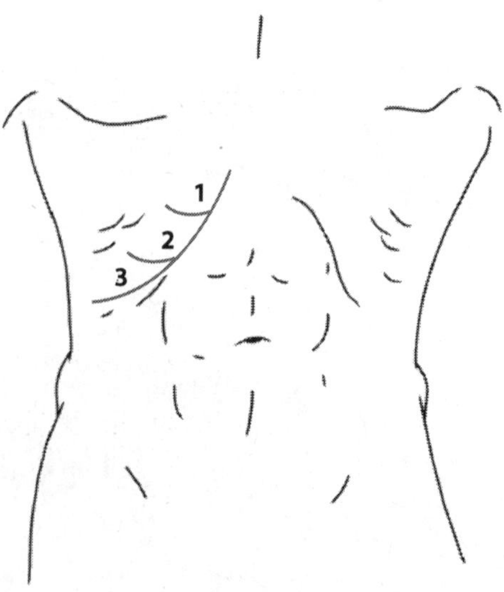

Figura 4.3 Diagnsis example

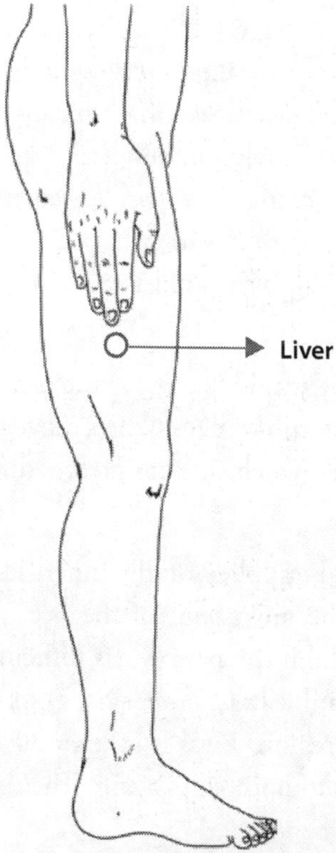

Figure 4.4 Point related to the liver in the leg

Treatment

With the person lying down with the tummy facing up, stretch the right arm along the body. The place where the middle finger of the hand touches the side of the leg is where the point related to the liver is located (see Figure 4.4).

Press this point at least 20 times with the thumb or, if it is very painful, with the palm of the hand. Each pressure should correspond to a breathe out.

Through touch, evaluate the condition of the liver again in the three points mentioned above in Figure 4.3. It should be better.

The ankles and neck

The ankles, in Japanese, are called *ashikubi,* which means "neck of the foot". The wrists are called *tekubi,* which means "neck of the hand". In *kanrenbui,* there is a direct relation between neck, ankles and wrists. We can say that the neck (of the head) is related to the neck of the foot (ankle) and to the neck of the hand (wrist). Therefore, the pains located in the neck can be treated in the ankles or wrists.

Diagnosis

The person must be sitting and move the head to both sides, making a bending movement with the neck. Each movement must be followed by a breathe out. Check which side has greater difficulty.

Treatment

The treatment will be applied on the inner side of the ankle contrary to the side in which the movement of the neck is harder, as shown in Figure 4.5. For example, if the person has difficulty to turn the neck to the right, treat the left ankle in its inner side. Look for a more painful and sensitive point in this region. Press it at least 20 times. Then check the movement of the neck to both sides again. The movement will be more fluid and the neck will be looser.

This point is very effective in treating stiff necks and pains in the neck in general. Mere bending movement or stretching of the wrists and ankles is indicated to relax the neck. We can sit and turn the ankles with the hands 30 times, at least, to each side; then we do the same with the wrists. Exercises that stretch the wrists and ankles, like some *yoga* poses, are also indicated.

When we have stiffness in the ankles or wrists or suffer from a lesion in these regions, we affect the condition of the neck. Likewise, a stiff condition of the neck causes certain vulnerability in the wrists and ankles.

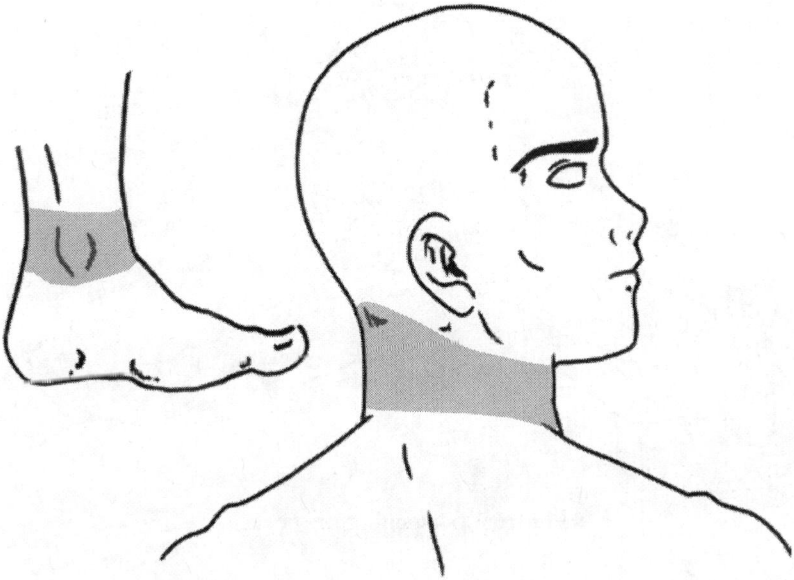

Figure 4.5 Relation of the ankle with the neck

Flexibility in opening the legs

The inner part of the legs is related to the inner part of the arms. Thus, people with little flexibility in opening the legs can be treated in the inner part of the arm.

Diagnosis

In this diagnosis, one must take the person's flexibility into account. We must measure the elastic capacity of the opening of the legs. Treatment is recommended if this is insufficient or unsatisfactory or when the person has pains in the inner part of the legs.

With the person sitting, with the legs stretched, ask him/her to open the legs as much as possible and check its opening, as shown in Figure 4.6.

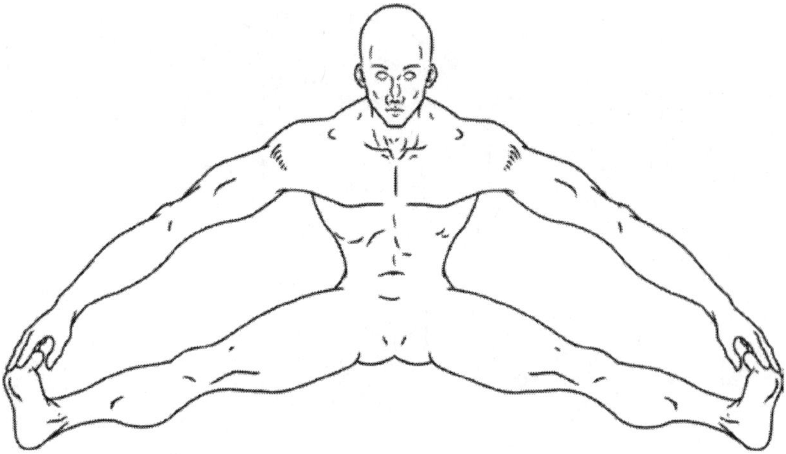

Figure 4.6 Opening of the legs

Treatment

With the person lying down with the tummy facing up, stimulate the anterior part of the arm, in the region between the armpit up to the elbow, pressing with the palm of the hand. Each pressure must be accompanied by a breathe out. Look in this region for the most sensitive or painful part and work it more. The treatment must be bilateral, that is, in both arms (see Figure 4.7).

Check the opening movement of the legs and check if there is increase in flexibility.

This treatment is very useful for gymnasts, athletes, martial arts and yoga practitioners, which are body works in which there is the need for great flexibility and opening of the legs.

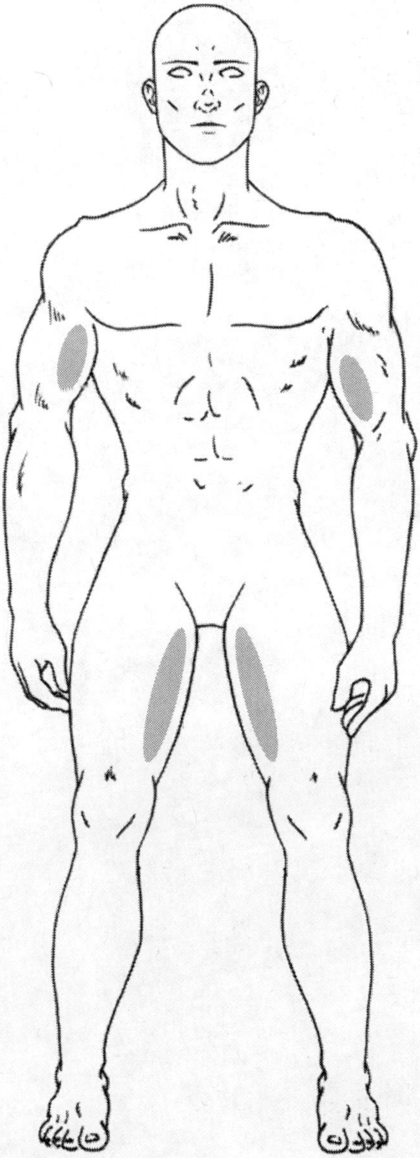

Figure 4.7 Relation of the arms with the legs

5

The hands

The hands have a direct relation with our mind. Note that in stressed, anxious, restless people, the hands shake and can have certain stiffness. In some people with much mental tension or serious mental problems, the hands become contracted, almost closed.

According to traditional Chinese medicine, hot hands mean very yang heart and mind, that is, they are overburdened. People with very hard and little flexible hands have a mind with this characteristic. A good massage in the hands calms us and makes us more balanced.

According to the kanrenbui method, our whole body is represented in the hands. The palm is related to the anterior part of the body, with the front part. The back is related to the posterior part of the body, the entire back part.

The outer fingers (thumbs and little fingers) are related to the legs. The ring fingers and index fingers are related to the arms and the middle fingers with the top part of the body: head and torso.

The palm of the hand is related to the abdomen and torso, with the back and kidneys.

We find in the hands points corresponding to all the joints of the body.

The spinal column is represented in the back of the hand, along the middle fingers.

The head is at the tip of the middle fingers. Therefore, in case of headache, we can stimulate the entire tip of the middle fingers. Look for the most sensitive point and stimulate it more.

The face is in the part of the flesh of the middle finger; there we find points to treat all problems of the face: there are points for the eyes, nose, mouth, throat, ears and teeth.

The manner of using these relations from kanrenbui is very simple. When the person (or we ourselves) has any complaint of pain or discomfort, we look in the hands for the point that is in the region related to the pain. This point will be very painful. We must press it 30 times or even until there is relief in the point of the hand.

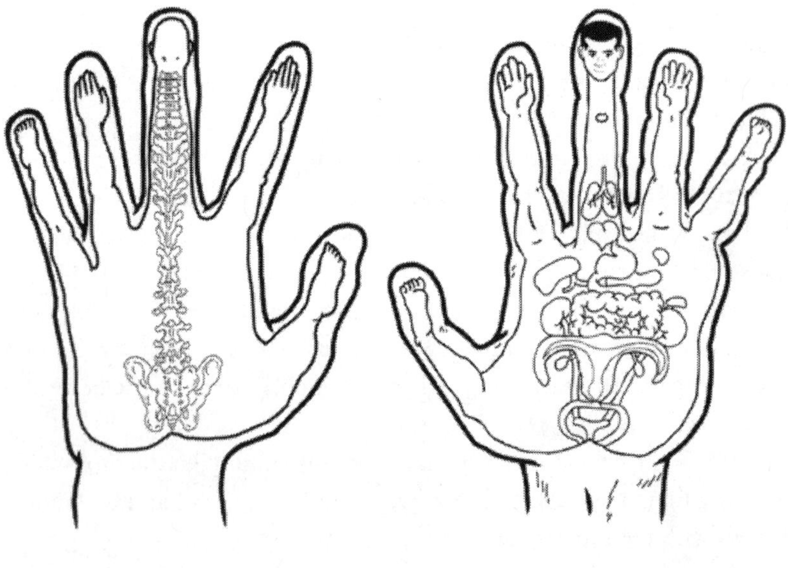

Figure 5.1 Representation of the body in the hands

Usually, it is more effective if we work the hand that is farther in relation to the place of pain in the body, however, one must stimulate the point in both hands. Stimulate a little in each hand and give greater attention to the more painful point.

The advantage of the points of the hands over the other points along the body is that they can easily be stimulated due to their location. They can be pressed several times a day. We can perform self-pressure and also teach the client to press himself.

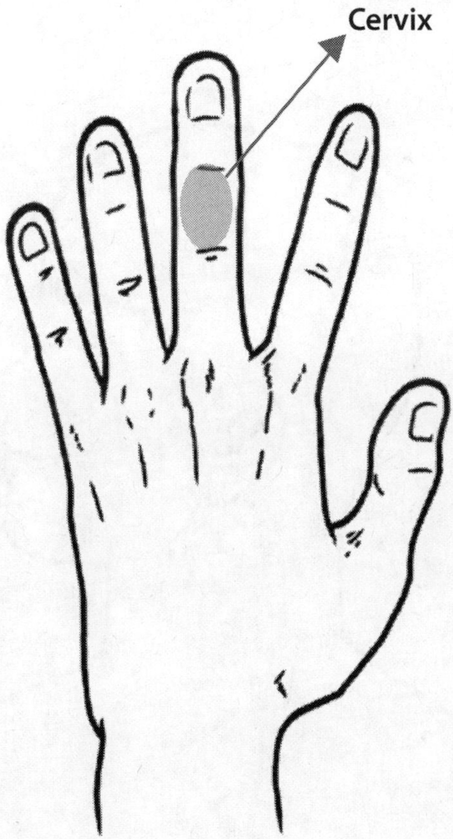

Figure 5.2 Relation of the cervical region in the hand

The cervical region and its representation in the hand

There is a direct relation between the neck and the second phalanx of the middle finger. This phalanx is also related to the cervical region of the spinal column, as shown in Figure 5.2. We can use this part in case of stiff neck, problems in the cervix, muscular pains in the nape or just tension in the nape and neck.

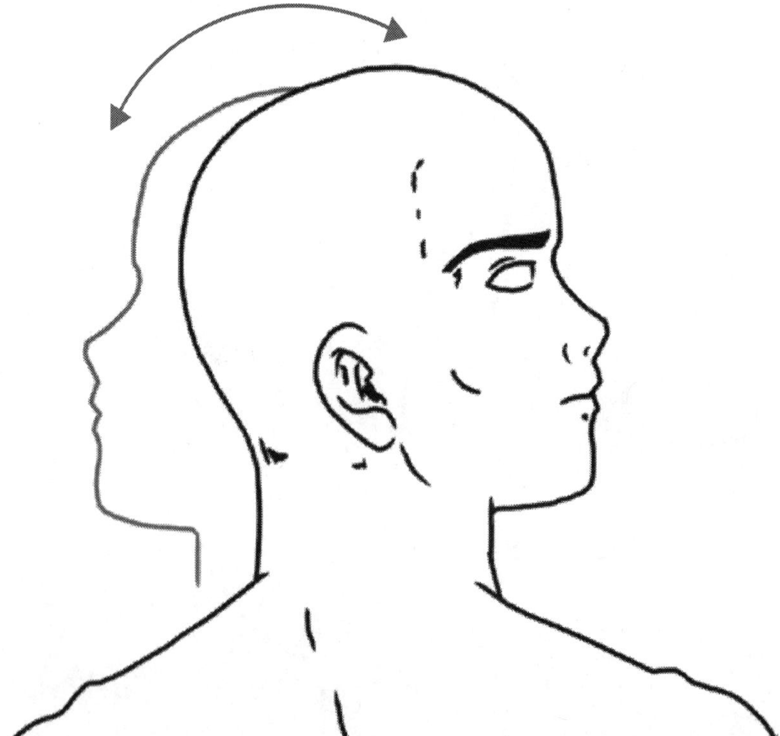

Figure 5.3 Bending of the cervix

Diagnosis

Move the head to both sides and identify the side to which there is greater difficulty in bending the neck: the right or left, as shown in Figure 5.3.

Treatment

The points related to this movement are found in the second phalanx of the middle finger (see Figure 5.2) and must be stimulated 30 times or until there is relief of the pain in the point pressed.

Check the bending movement of the neck again and you will see an improvement, especially on the side in which the movement was stiffer.

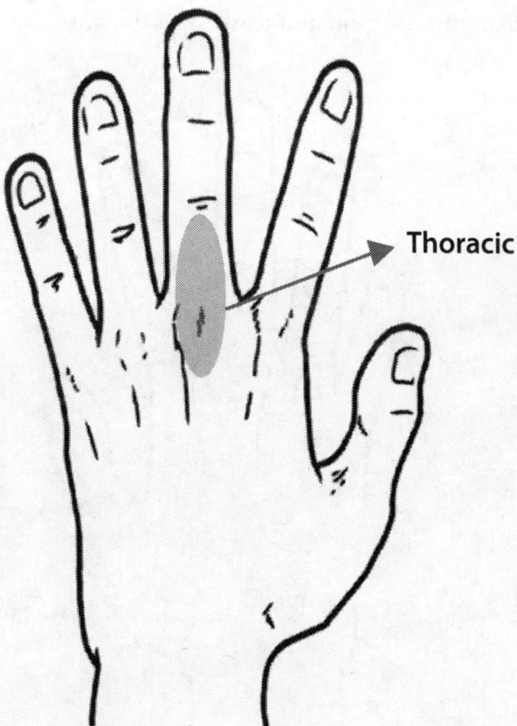

Figure 5.4 Relation of the thoracic region in the hand

The thoracic region and its representation in the hand

On the back of the hand, we can find points related to the thoracic vertebrae of the spine. In the top part of the back of the hand, we find an area corresponding to the thoracic cavity. This area covers the beginning of the middle finger and the top part of the back of the hand.

When the person has pain or tension in the musculature of the dorsal region, there may be a problem in the spinal column in this region, such as scoliosis, or cyphosis. We can identify this region in both hands and find the more painful point. We must then treat it as already mentioned previously and check the place of tension or problem in the back, checking for an improvement and relaxing of the musculature.

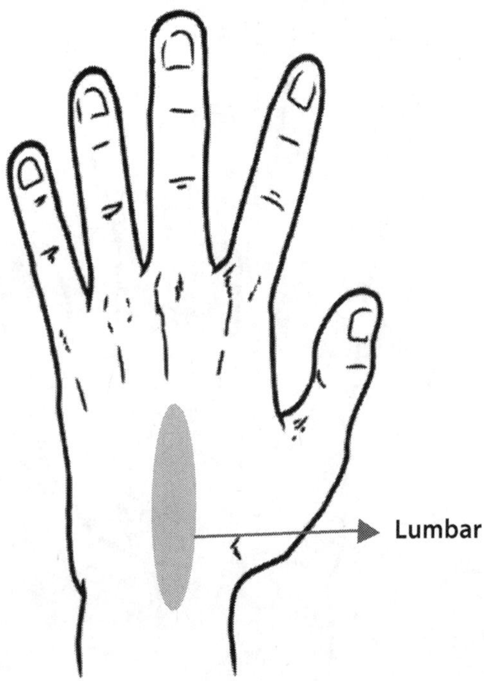

Figure 5.5 Relation of the lumbar region in the hand

The lumbar region and its representation in the hand

The middle part of the back of the hand up to the wrist is related to the lumbar and sacral re-gion. The area related to the coccyx is located in a depression in the middle of the wrist. This entire part in the back of the hand is very efficient for the treatment of muscular pains in the lumbar region, pains in the sciatic nerve, disk hernias, protrusions and other symptoms. This region is also related to the kidneys. We must look for the related points in both hands and treat the more painful.

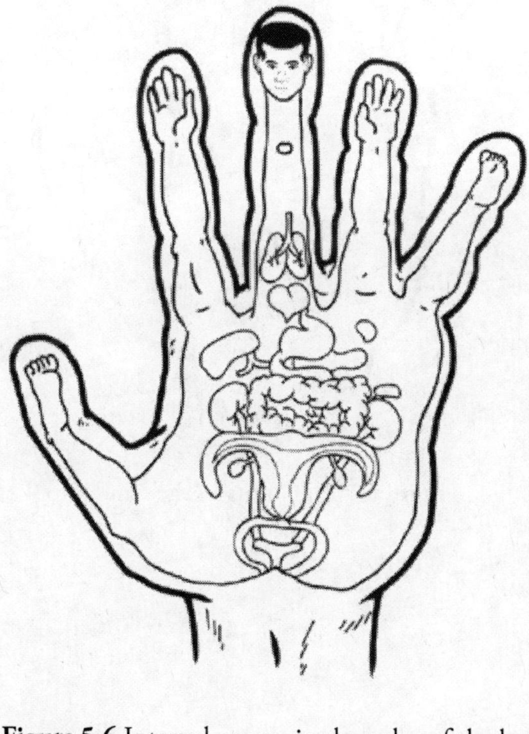

Figure 5.6 Internal organs in the palm of the hand

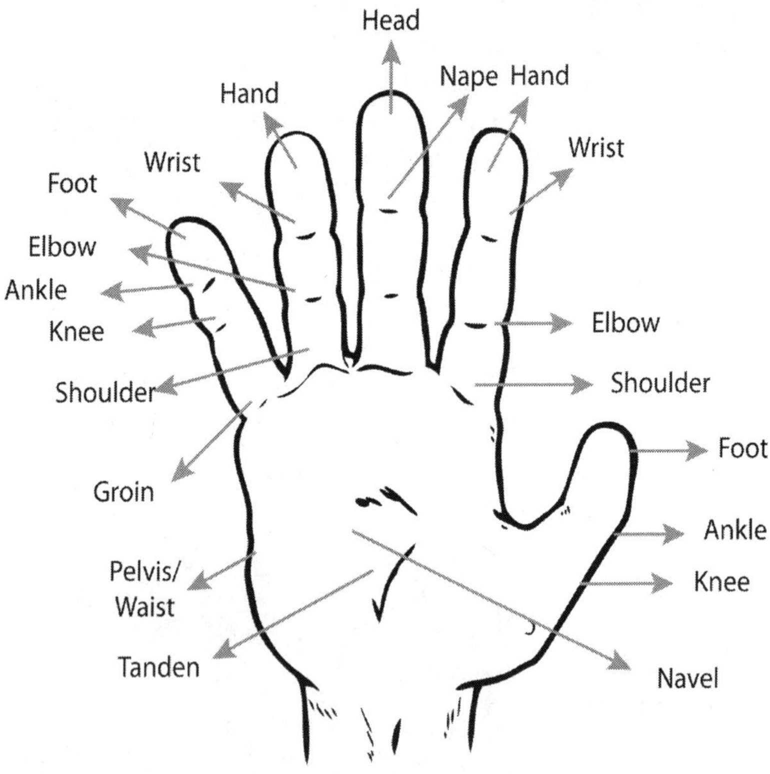

Figure 5.7 The joints in the hand

Internal organs and the palm of the hand

The palm of the hand is related to the internal organs. Pains or digestive problems can be treated in it efficiently.

Diagnosis

Make an organic diagnosis through touch. By slowly and deeply pressing the abdomen with the fingers of both hands together, check the region that is stiffest and/or with the most pain.

Treatment

Look in the palm of both hands for the point related to this region. Press it with the thumb and check in which hand it is more painful. Give greater attention to the more painful hand, pressing the point at least 30 times.

Next, check the region of the abdomen again. You will note that there was a relaxing of the tension in this region and relief of the pain. Naturally, if there is an imbalance or disease in the internal organ, this treatment must be done daily or with the highest possible frequency.

The joints and their representation in the hand

As we can see in Figure 5.7, each one of the joints of the fingers is related to the joints of the arms and legs. All the joints of the body are represented in the hand.

For example, the front or anterior part of the knees is related to the front or anterior part of the finger joint. The inner side of the knee corresponds to the joint of the finger and the outer part of the finger is related to the outer side of the knee.

In the joint of the finger, with the back of the hand, we find points related to the shoulders and areas of the trapezius. There, we can treat pains in the shoulders and tension in the trapezius.

6

The arms

Point related to the liver

In the posterior part of the arm, above the right elbow, there is a very effective point to treat the liver. In cases of excessive consumption of alcohol or medical drugs or when the person is receiving chemotherapy treatment, the functions of the liver are compromised, the organ is overburdened. In this case, the use of this point is very beneficial.

Diagnosis

In the region of the liver, in the top part on the right side of the abdomen, press three points to check if there is stiffness and/or pain in any of them, as shown in Figure 6.2.

Treatment

Press with the thumb the point above the elbow. One can also use moxibustion (heating of the point with moxa stick) in this point in cases where the liver is increased in size or with accumulation of fat.

Check the region of the liver again in the abdomen and check if there was a relief in the stiffness or pain in the organ.

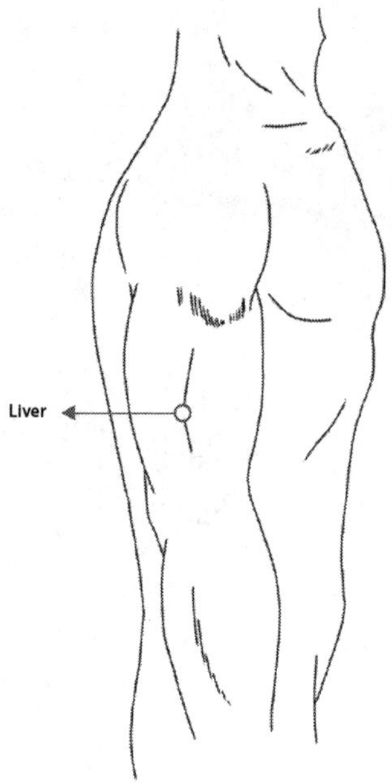

Figure 6.1 Point related to the liver in the arm

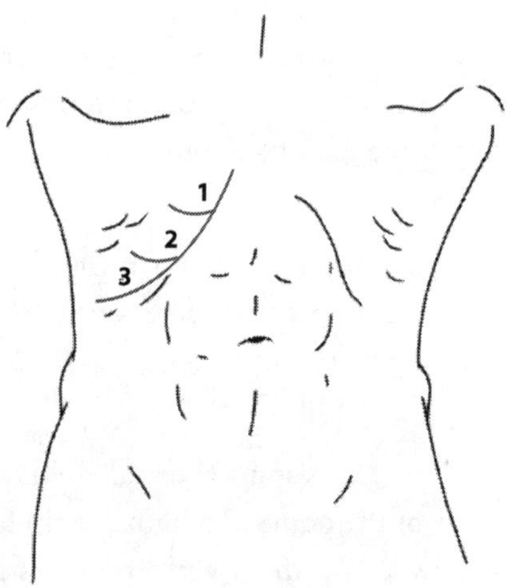

Figure 6.2 Diagnosis of the liver region

Solar plexus, breathing and corresponding part in the arm

In the region of the arm with the forearm, near the elbow, we find a relation with the region of the solar plexus, where there is the liver, gall-bladder, stomach, spleen and pancreas, the organs that are located in the upper part of the abdomen, as shown in Figure 6.3.

When we stimulate this region, there is a relaxation in these organs, causing an improvement in breathing, since breathing is shorter when these organs are too tense. When the person has respiratory problems, we press this area with the palm of the hand and rub strongly from the center outwards, in this entire region, as shown in Figure 6.4.

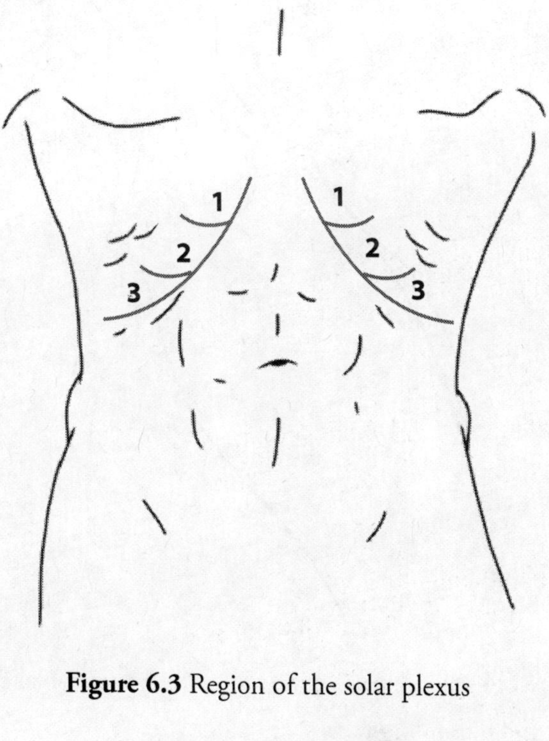

Figure 6.3 Region of the solar plexus

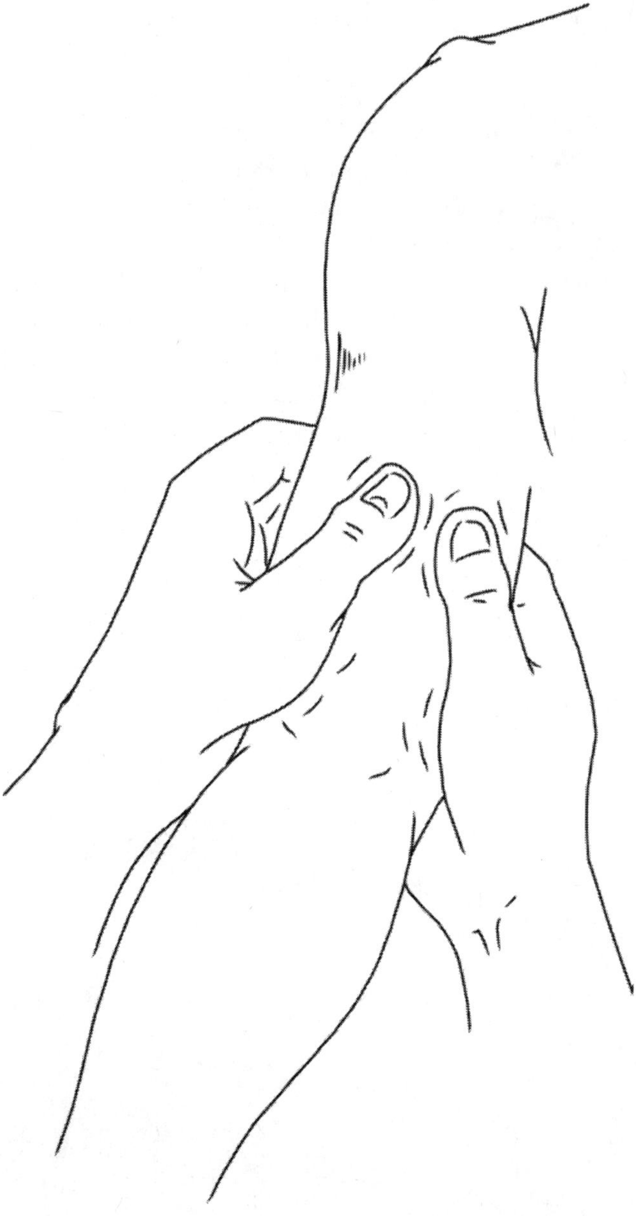

Figure 6.4 Middle part of the arm related to the solar plexus

Points related to the trapezius

In the beginning of the arm, in its anterior side, we find three very efficient points to treat the trapeze muscle on the same side of the arm. We can use these points in cases of stiff neck, strong stiffness or muscular tension in the trapezius.

The trapezius, in the area of the shoulders, becomes very stiff, especially when the person has constipation, suffers from hypertension and when the body's energy is located more in the top part. In general, people with much mental activity and practice little physical activity have no force in the *tanden,* the physical and energy center of the body, accumulate more tension in the region of the shoulders.

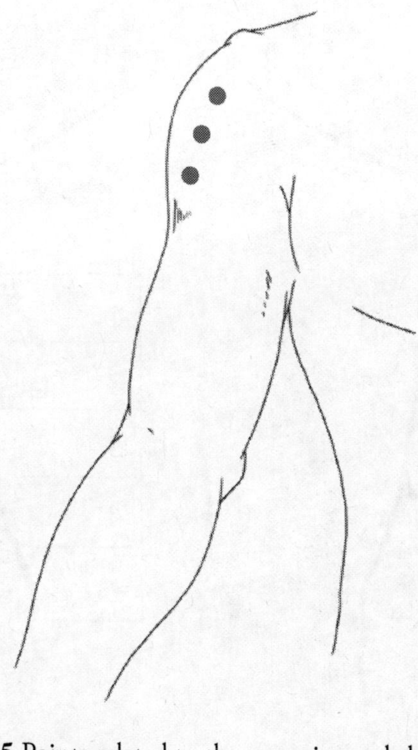

Figure 6.5 Points related to the trapezius and shoulders

Diagnosis

With the person sitting, ask him/her to turn a shoulder, making circular movements to and fro. Ask him/her to do the same with the other shoulder. Check which of them has the stiffer movement.

Treatment

With the person lying down or sitting, press the three points in the arm with circular movements, the points are shown in Figure 6.5. Identify the most painful point out of the three and press it more times. Check the circular movement of both shoulders again. You will see that the shoulder that was stiffer will be looser, making the movement more easily. This point should be used when the person has strong pain or tension in the shoulder and in the trapezius.

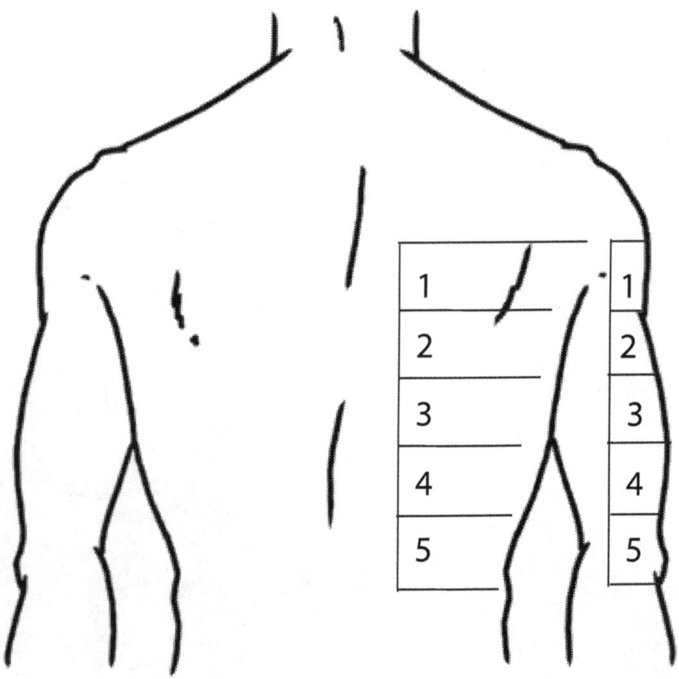

Figure 6.6 Points in the arm related to the back

Points for the musculature of the back (paravertebral)

Tensions and pains in the paravertebral muscles must be treated in the arm. We must identify the point of pain and, from there, trace an imaginary line up to the arm of the same side. With the palm of the hand facing the body, we look for the point in the posterior part of the arm, always at the height corresponding to the pain in the back, as shown in Figure 6.6.

Pains or tensions in the dorsal region, between the scapulae and spinal column, are very common, especially in breastfeeding mothers, due to the increased weight of the breasts and weight of the baby. Also, people who stay for long periods in front of the computer, using one arm more than the other, usually feel these pains. Treating the corresponding point in the arm, at the height of the pain, is very efficient.

Treatment

Press this region in the top and posterior part of the arm of the same side in which there is pain. Identify the most painful point in the arm at the same height as the back pain (see Figure 6.6). Press it with the thumb about 30 times, in coordination with the expiration. Check the region where there was pain or tension again. Check if the musculature is more relaxed.

7

The spinal column

The spinal column has a triple importance: physical, mental and organic. Pains in the paravertebral musculatures, symptoms related to the vertebrae, scoliosis, cyphosis, hyperlordosis and disk hernias, among so many others, show not only a physical impairment, but also mental and organic disorders.

According to traditional Chinese medicine, the meridian of the governing vessel is located in the spinal column. This meridian is related to the central nervous system; therefore, we can say that problems in the nervous system directly affect the position of the spinal column, affecting our posture. People who have shoulders displaced forward indicate, besides a postural problem, a possible depression and introverted personality. Other symptoms, like lumbar pains, are related to digestive problems and malfunctioning of the sexual organs.

Each one of the vertebrae is related to an organic function. Thus, a pain in the spine does not only indicate a problem in the vertebra, but also a disorder in the related organic part. In the Oki-Do method, there are many exercises aimed at correcting posture, consequently improving the organic functions. The countless points shown here—in the arms, hands and legs—also generate these benefits to the posture and related organic function.

The pains located in the spinal column or in the spiny processes of the vertebrae can indicate psychic problems, emotional and psychological stress, in this case influencing or being influenced by the central nervous system (see Figure 7.1). The treatments with moxibustion are very effective in the vertebrae and have a more immediate result, but one can also press with the fingers the points related to the vertebrae in the feet and hands, improving the condition in this region of the spinal column and in the organ related to it.

Tracing an imaginary vertical line two centimeters from the spinal column, where the paravertebral muscles are located, one will find a region that is related to the organs (see Figure 7.1).

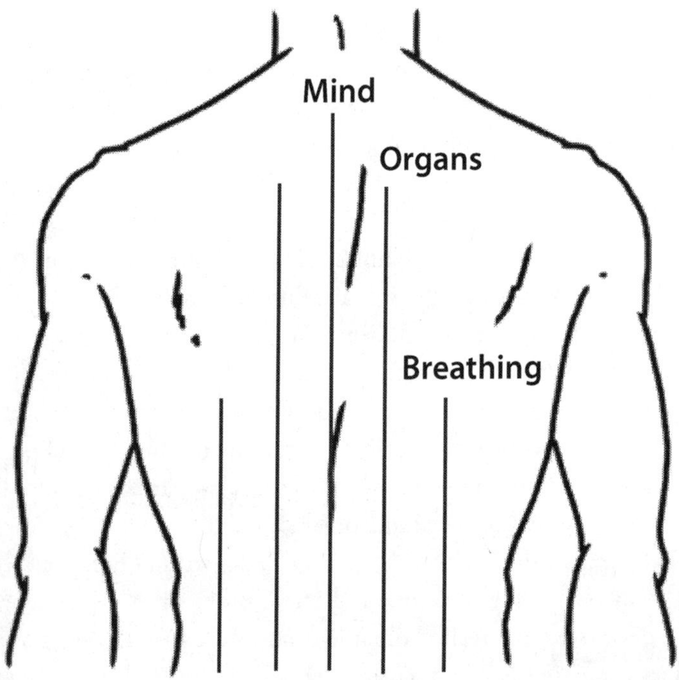

Figure 7.1 Relation of the back with the mind, organs and breathing

Pains or tensions located in this region indicate an organic imbalance.

According to the western concept of medicine, muscular pains in the back are caused by bad posture or excess physical effort, like carrying something heavy, etc.

According to the oriental concept, specifically according to the precepts of Masahiro Oki, the pains in the posterior musculature of the back are always related to an organic imbalance. Therefore, we should not focus only on treating the region of the back where the pain is located. For an effective treatment, we must focus our attention on treating the organ related to the region that has pain.

A third line from the lower point of the scapula up to the hip is associated with difficulty in the respiratory part, as shown in Figure 7.1. Pain, tension or stiffness in this region indicates a type of respiratory problem. When we treat this region through pressure with the fingers and with the hands, there is an improvement in breathing.

The spine in relation to the internal organs

As we described in the chapter on internal organs, many pains in the spine are associated with an organic malfunctioning. In the thoracic region, we find relations with the lung and heart. According to oriental medicine, these organs are related to the emotions. When the person shows emotional imbalance, he/she usually has bad posture and his/her thoracic region is more curved to the front.

The middle part of the thoracic region is related to the organs of the solar plexus, stomach, spleen, pancreas, liver and gallbladder. Malfunctioning of these organs can cause tension in the paravertebral musculature or even scoliosis. These organs must be treated to improve the person's posture.

The low part of the thoracic region, the lumbar and sacral regions are related to the large and small intestines, with the bladder and sexual organs. Tension in this area can cause a bending of the pelvis, causing symptoms like menstrual cramps or intestinal malfunctioning.

See the relations between organs and the spine in Figure 7.2.

Relation of the vertebrae

The *ka*nrenbui method treats the person holistically: the changes and pains in the vertebrae of the spine indicate a problem in the spine itself, but also an organic, respiratory, psychic and/or emotional imbalance. We must therefore treat the vertebra in the related points found in the hands, feet and also in the points related to the internal organs. One must also take care of the diet, practicing a more balanced and healthy diet. The respiratory part must also be improved through frequent physical activities and specific breathing exercises. We must also develop our ability to adapt to the changes and difficulties of life. When we improve the spine, we also improve our adaptability: flexibility of the spine causes greater mental flexibility.

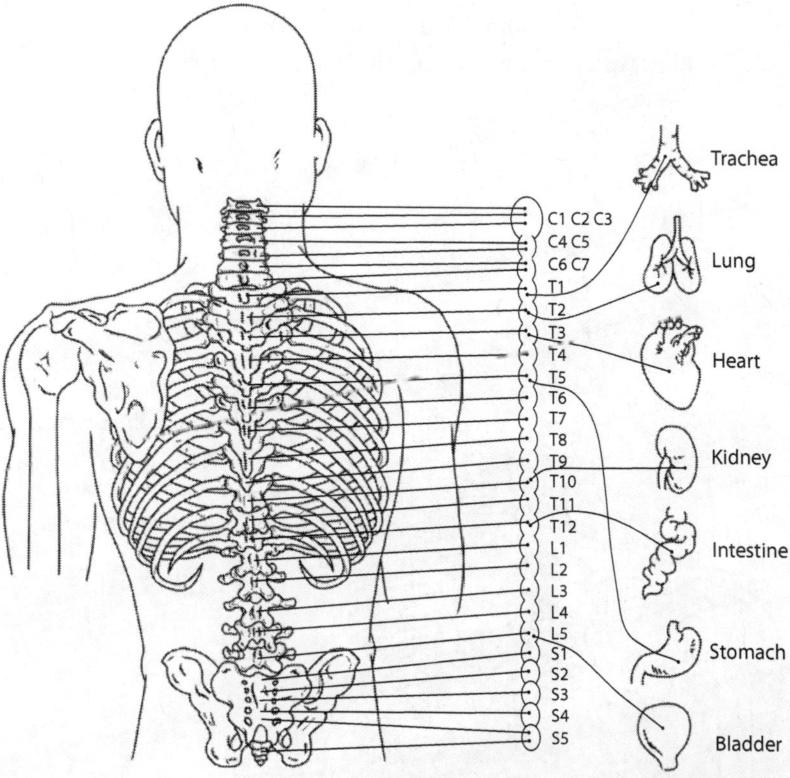

Figure 7.2 Relation of the spine with the internal organs

Cervical vertebrae

The illustrations below show us the relations of each vertebra.

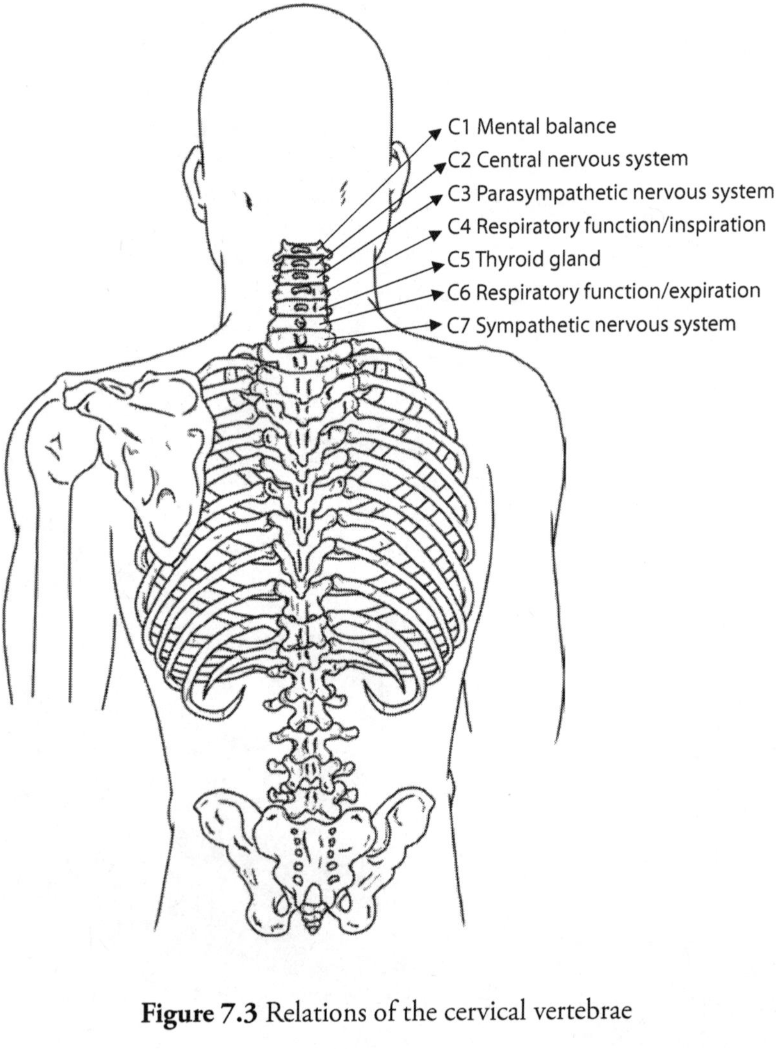

Figure 7.3 Relations of the cervical vertebrae

Thoracic vertebrae

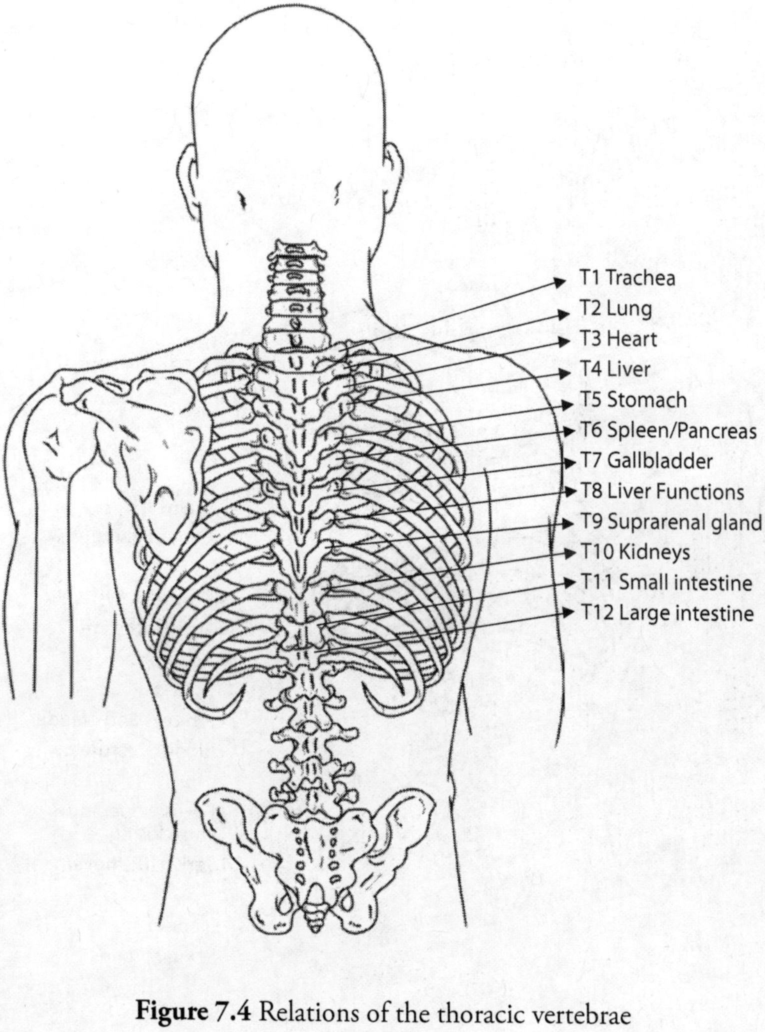

Figure 7.4 Relations of the thoracic vertebrae

Lumbar vertebrae

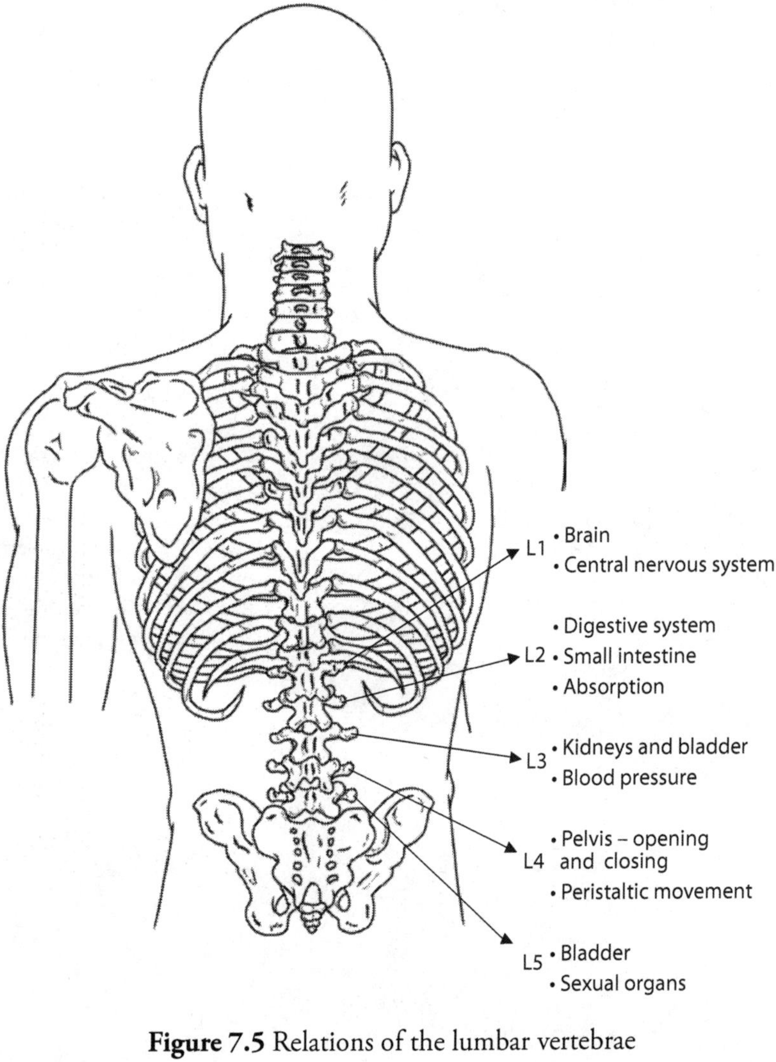

Figure 7.5 Relations of the lumbar vertebrae

Sacral vertebrae

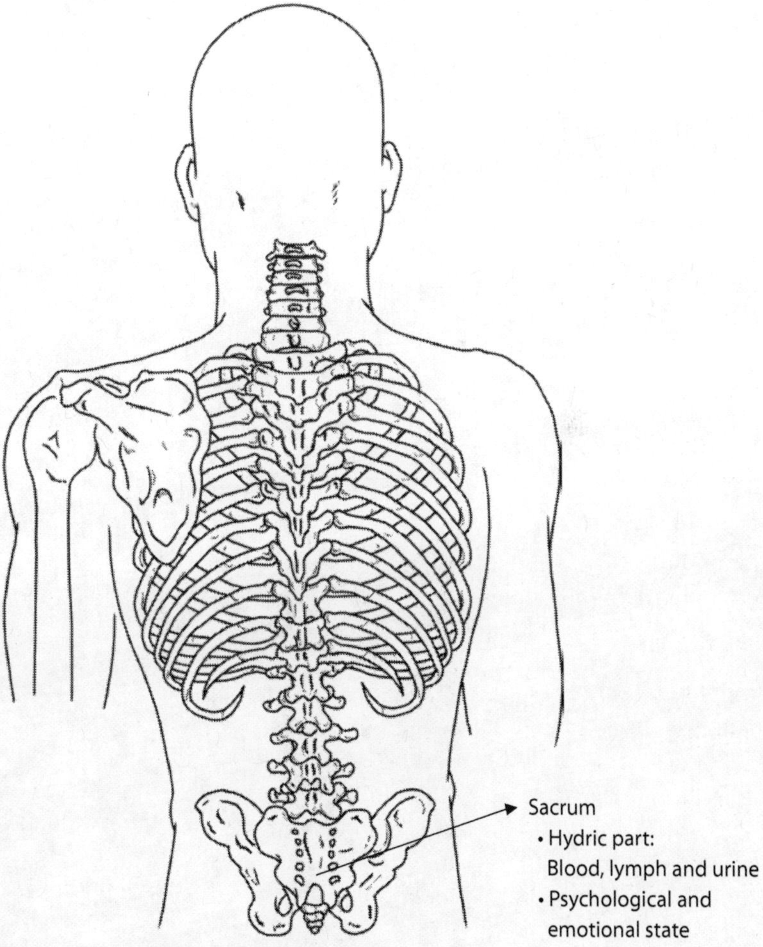

Figure 7.6 Relations of the sacral vertebrae

8

The thoracic cavity

The thoracic cavity is directly related to breathing. In the Oki-Do method, there are certain exercises that develop the musculature, making the thoracic cavity more flexible, increasing respiratory capacity, which is fundamental for good health and quality of life.

In the thoracic cavity, we find a series of points connected to the senses (smell, sight, hearing and taste), as shown in Figure 8.1. When the chest is contracted, these functions are affected.

Exercises that expand the thoracic cavity are also important to improve these senses.

Hearing

In the lateral part of the thoracic cavity, in the anterior serratus muscle, we find a point related to hearing, as shown in Figure 8.1. Ear problems always indicate sensitivity or pain in these points in the thoracic cavity. In cases of buzzing in the ear or hearing loss, stimulate the point of the same side, at least 30 times, everyday.

Sight

The sides of the sternum, in the upper part of the thoracic cavity, are related to sight.

There is an exercise that clearly shows how to use these points: cover one eye with the hand and check the sight of the other, focusing on an object in front. Do the same with the other eye. Identify which of them sees the object less. Myopic people should focus on a distant object and people with tired sight can focus on reading a nearer text. Check which eye sees less and stimulate the corresponding thorax area, on the same side. On finding the most sensitive point in this region, press it 30 times. Then check the sight of each eye again separately. The eye on the same side in which the point was stimulated will have a better sight than before.

For people with sight problems, we must press both sides of the sternum (see Figure 8.1), together with the points for sight mentioned in chapter 2 on the head (see Figures 2.8 and 2.9).

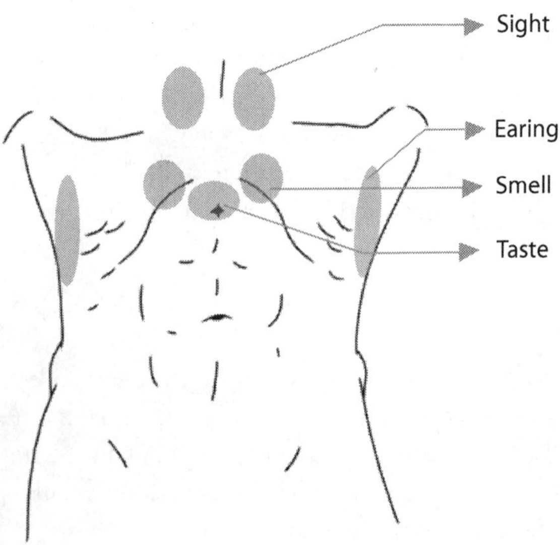

Figure 8.1 Parts related to the organs of the senses in the thoracic cavity

Smell

The sides of the ribs, beside the sternum bone, in the region below the nipples, are related to the nasal cavities. The area on the right side of the thorax corresponds to the right nostril and the left area corresponds to the left nostril (see Figure 8.1). Also, the internal organs on the right side of the abdomen are related with the right nostril. And the internal organs on the left side are related with the right nostril.

The right nostril corresponds to the more yang part of the body and the left nostril to the more yin part.

We use these points to unblock the nostrils and improve smell. When a nostril has difficulty to inhale and exhale, we press the points of the same side of the nostril in the thorax.

Check which side of the nose is blocked and stimulate the corresponding point at least 30 times. The nostril will unblock quickly, facilitating breathing. Pressure in these points also stimulates the sense of smell.

Taste

The end of the sternum bone, in the region we usually call mouth of the stomach, is related to the mouth and taste (see Figure 8.1). We must stimulate this region when the person has problems of acidity or loss of taste.

9

Inochi

Order, command, mission, life, soul

The human being is not only physical, but is also a manifestation of an internal and external process. As breathing, organic functions, diet, thought influenced by the environment that we live. Therefore, the manifestation of symptoms and diseases in our body are the natural expression of our inner force, Inochi. They are as messages, or warnings of our inner force, telling us that something is not well.

For the oriental philosophy, Inochi governs all mind and body functions, as motion, reproduction, absorption, elimination, sleep, thought, etc.

Inochi, our inner force, is our ally and protector, it tries to balance us. A lot of times our diseases, pains, or a simple alteration of our physical posture is a warning of our inner force, telling us that we are not acting correctly with our body or with our being.

Inochi is intimately linked with our unconscious, with our essence, with the most intimate part of our being.

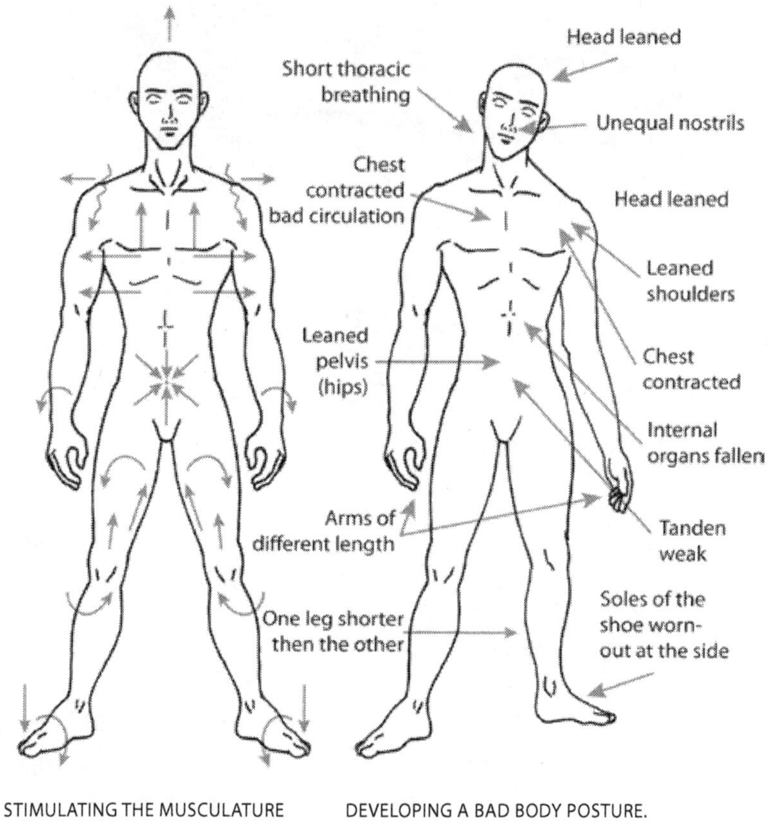

Figure 9.1 Natural Balanced Posture

Breathing influences our Inochi. When we keep a deep and natural breathing, we can harmonize our Inochi.

Natural and balanced posture

There are several reasons why our physical body change, causing unbalance in our natural posture, such as:

- Bad organic functions, sedentary life, lack of body moviment, repetitive movements, negative thoughts, attached emotions.

Knowing that the thought and organic functions change our physical posture, we can work to restore our posture improving our thought and our organic functions (see Figure 9.2).

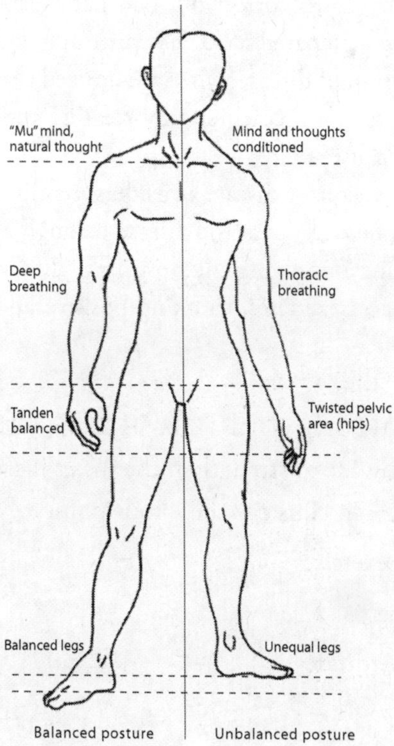

Figure 9.2 our thoughts and habits influence our physical posture

Our Inochi, inner force, express all physical and mental changes of our being.

Our habits can modify our natural physical posture, that's why we need corrective exercises, through them we strengthened our "good and pure" side and corrected the "defective" side.

We improve not only the physical part, but also our behavior, thoughts, emotions, this way making a better use of our potentiality in daily life.

In the Orient, during our studies we heard this sentence several times "Your disease is your master", at first it seems hard to accept, but then, through ours and the others′ experience, we understood that the pain, the disease teaches us to correct our bad habits, to have healthier attitudes, to eat better prepared food that suits our body health condition. In the western vision of disease, when we noticed that we are sick or have a pain, soon we take a medicine, only treating the symptoms and not caring about the cause.

The oriental vision of disease considers mainly the cause, considers our inner part, intends to treat the disease through changing habits, correcting the posture, improving the breathing, diet, elimination, making appropriate physical exercises, thinking positive and improving mental attitude before life.

Strengthen the inner force

There are several ways to strengthen the inner force turning it more a live. Basically we can consider these four points:

- Physical exercises
- Breathing
- Mental Attitude
- Diet

Physical exercise

Our body gets habits in daily life; we use the same muscles in a repetitive way, according to our work circumstances. It can work out a group of muscles and atrophy others that are not being used. In this case our inner force shows us that something is wrong through pains and body posture changes, for instance a twist on the hips. Through the corrective exercises, we can restore these unbalances correcting the posture and improving the flexibility.

As we are working our body, we understand that strengthen the Tanden is essential to increase flexibility in the superior part of the body and strengthen the musculature of the lower part of the body, that should be connected to the ground. This way we attain balance in the body.

If we observe nature, the wild animals, for instance, reestablish their own balance alone. They don't go to the veterinarian, nor they use any special medicine, they heal themselves with what their natural habitat has to offer them. In Japan, it is called "monpo", this self cure inner force is the manifestation of the vital force. The human being also has this internal wisdom, this instinct, and it can be rescued and strengthened through corrective exercises, fast and faith.

Exercises to strengthen the inner force

Physical posture: seating in seiza, as shown in Figure 9.3, with your hands palms together, on chest's height, symbolizing unity and prayer, keeping the column erect and shoulders relaxed.

Breathing: breathe deep and natural, feeling the abdomen to expand while you inhale and to contract, to empty while you exhale.

Mental posture: concentrate on Tanden. Cultivate in your heart a soft feeling of gratitude.

Although doing only a few minutes of this practice daily, it will bring you a balance and well being sensation.

Seating in "seiza 'doing' gassho"

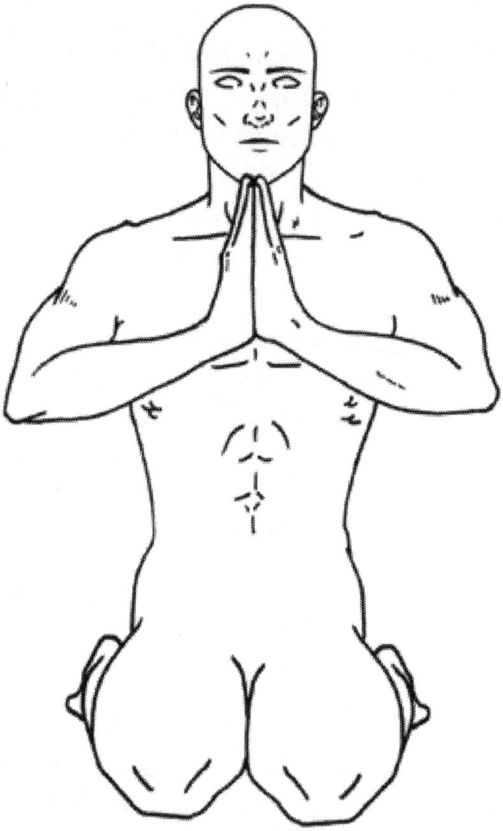

Figure 9.3 Gassho Posture

Breathing

Our breath should be deep and abdominal, in other words, when inhaling the abdomen expands and when exhaling the abdomen contracts. The exhalation time should last twice as the inhalation.

Through a good breathing we can assimilate the "pneuma" as it's called by the Greeks, "prana" as it's called by the Hindus , "chi" by the Chinese and "ki" by the Japanese, in English we can call it "life blow".

A deep and balanced breathing produces a better emotional balance, better mental concentration, and an appropriate physical relaxation, increasing our being's capacity in all ways.

Through thoracic breathing the air reaches only the superior part of the lungs. And the exhalation does not eliminate completely the air contained in our lungs, prevent the complete renew of the air in the lungs. This kind of breathing is more common when we are tense or anxious. The muscles of the superior part of the body are more rigid, increasing the tension level in the shoulders.

If we pay attention to a recently born child, days or months old, when he/she is sleeping, we can observe the perfect movement of his/her abdomen,

when inhaling inflates the abdomen and when exhaling empties the abdomen. Natural breathing is like this, very simple. Even though most people, in the adult age, doesn't breathe naturally due to accumulated tension on the thorax and shoulders area. This can bring physical and emotional problems for the person's health.

Breathing practice to increase ours "life blow"

Posture: lying on your back, legs bent knees together and feet leaning on the ground, see in Figure 9.4.

Breathing: inhale deep and slowly expanding your abdomen without dilating your nostrils. Paying more attention to the exhalation, that should last twice of the inhalation time. Try to exhale the air of the lungs completely.

For instance, you can mentally count up to 4 inhaling, and up to 8 exhaling, until this breathing rhythm becomes natural and you no longer need to count.

Stay breathing for 5 minutes approximately.

Breathe approximately for 5 minutes.

Place your hands, or even a book, on your abdomen to feel its ascendant and descendent movement.

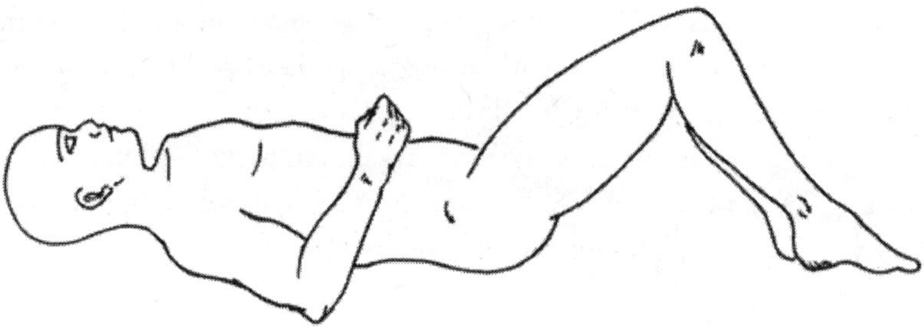

Figure 9.4 Posture to practice deep breathing

Diet to strengthen Inochi

A balanced diet, with organic cereals, vegetables and organic green vegetables, is what our organism needs for an appropriate functioning.

We should consume food of the season, in other words, considering eating fruits and vegetables of the season.

Summer time we should eat more fruits, salads and raw vegetables. Due to the heat of the season, the organism needs colder food that contains more liquid to cool of our body. That is very important for the heart balance, which is the organ that is more sensitive in this season.

In the winter, it is necessary to ingest hotter and stronger food, as roots and cooked cereals, reducing the amount of fruits. These roots and cooked cereals benefit the kidneys and the lungs, which are the organs that feel more difficulty in this season.

It is also important to consume more food from the region we live. As in Brazil, a tropical country, we should consume more fruits and green vegetables. Though in a cold climate country, we should consume more animal products and less fruits.

In general a balanced meal consists of consuming 50% of whole grain cereals and 50% divided among roots, vegetables, green vegetables, fruits and some animal products. This is what we call a balanced meal.

The whole grain cereals were the base of the diet of all the ancient people. In the Far East the base of their diet was rice, in the Middle East nuts and semolina, in Europe wheat and in America corn.

The cereal should be the human being's main food. It is ideal for humans, because its proportion between sodium and potassium is very similar to the proportion found in the man's blood, and also on animals that are fed with cereals.

The cereal should be whole, the whole grain, because it is at the external part of the grain that we find most of vitamins and minerals, and also the fibers necessary for our organism

Practical experience with whole grain rice

- In an open container (a glass or a jar), put some moisten cotton (with water), and put on top some grains of raw whole grain rice.
- In another container do the same procedure, but use white rice grains.
- Moisten the cotton everyday with a little bit of water.

Around the 3rd and the 5th day you will notice that the whole grain rice sprouted, you will see a new plant, and that the white rice deteriorated.

This happens because the whole grain rice still has in its grain the germ that creates a new plant, it has vital force, it has life and can bring more life to our organism. In the other hand the white rice doesn't have life in its grain, when it was refined its germ was removed, it was also removed the vitamins, minerals, and the fibers of its grain.

We should try to eat vegetables, fruits and green vegetables without chemicals, without pesticides. The purest food, more natural has its vital force stronger than the polluted ones, with chemical products.

In Korea they made a very interesting experiment about that. There is a very energetic root called ginseng, to consume this root can improve our physical strength, it has many therapeutic uses. This root should be picked after 3 years of been planted, after 3 years of life below the soil. As there was an excessive increase in the consumption of the ginseng, the Koreans began to use chemical fertilizers so that it could develop more quickly and could be pulled of the soil in less time. However they verified that the ginseng being planted this way lost their therapeutic uses. Then the scientists began to study these roots, and they compare them with the other one planted without fertilizers, they found the same nutrients and in the same proportions. They concluded that the difference between the roots was on the time they stayed buried. The ginseng kept buried for 3 years in the soil, had a stronger vital force than the one that was less time under the soil. The root with more vital force had larger therapeutic effects than the other.

In the same way, the vegetables, green vegetables and organic fruits, cultivated without chemical products, have more vitality acquired from the earth, the sun, and the water. This vitality is transferred to those that consume them.

Fast food, industrialized food, tin can food and the frozen ones are chaotic for our organism, because they have a large amount of preservative and other chemistries noxious to our body.

Alcoholic drinks, soft drinks and food that contains white sugar, should be avoided or consumed in small amounts. All these foods help to eliminate important minerals of our organism, increasing the free radicals and letting our body vulnerable to diseases and accelerating the aging process.

Mental attitude

Our mind influences directly our body, and a lot of times modify him. We should always think positive, because it encourages our immunological and organic system to function better.

For instance, if we think that we are with our energy low, and we begin to repeat this thought constantly, "I am so tired", this can become reality or can make our fatigue worse.

The symptoms and anomalies presented by our body are not always fixed, our body is in a constant transformation, life is constantly changing, and the Universe is in a constant movement. It is an illusion to think that things have stopped, or that they seem always the same. The planet Earth rotates around its own axis, and at the same time around the Sun, the solar system moves inside of the Milky Way, that moves in the Universe. Likewise our body, as part of all this, is full of cycles and changes.

When our thoughts become fixed, attached in some symptom, it can worsen our condition or make us sick. For instance, when somebody tells you that your liver condition is not well, and you fix your thoughts in this diagnosis and then worry too much about this, you will be creating favorable conditions for your liver really not work well. On the other hand if you take a positive attitude towards this diagnosis, listening to your inner force, looking for a more appropriate diet for your liver, as to eat more green color and sour flavored food. Stimulate the points related to the liver, and mainly, watch what is causing you such altered humors and emotions, as a bad mood and anger, because these feelings influence the functions of the liver. This is a mental attitude of occupy with the fact and not of preoccupy.

We needed to have clear the difference between to occupy and to preoccupy with things that could happen to us, most of the time they don't even happen. Worries affect the good function of the stomach.

To have a positive mental attitude in relation to a diagnosis is to occupy with it, it is to learn how to treat this symptoms, to go on a better diet, to change the attitude towards the problems and difficulties that life presents us. It is also to cultivate positive thoughts, to learn to forgive who hurt us, to forgive ourselves from our own mistakes. It is to have faith, to ask for help when needed and, also to help the nearest ones; it is to give attention to our relationships, enjoying it; improve our physical activities, in short, to look for a healthier life.

To worry and to think only about the disease, to foment cata-strophic expectations, to repeat to oneself "I can't", "I am not able to", to be closed for changes, to complain and to mutter, all this leaks our vital force, it weaken our being and we lose our inner force of cure, of rebalance.

A lot of people carry a diagnosis for many years as if it was their cross. But if one had had a more positive attitude towards to the symptoms, their organism could had already changed its condition.

Our inner force knows what is good for our body, for our health. We need to learn to always listen to our inner force.

Practice of the influence of the mental attitude on the physical body:

- Posture: Standing up, bend the column forward, try to reach the floor, without bending your knees, as show in Figure 9.5.
- Due to rigidity in the lumbar area, most people can't reach the ground.
- Back on the standing posture, close your eyes and imagine that you are a jelly. Then, move your body to all sides, as if you really were a jelly, without rigidity, boneless.
- Inhaling and exhaling slowly, imagine a jelly when you take it out of the refrigerator, this jelly is you. Move you body continuously liberating it from all tensions.

- Open your eyes, and again bend your body forward trying to reach the ground. You will fell your body more flexible, and that you can even touch the ground.

Through this practice, we noticed that the thought and the imagination can directly influence the body.

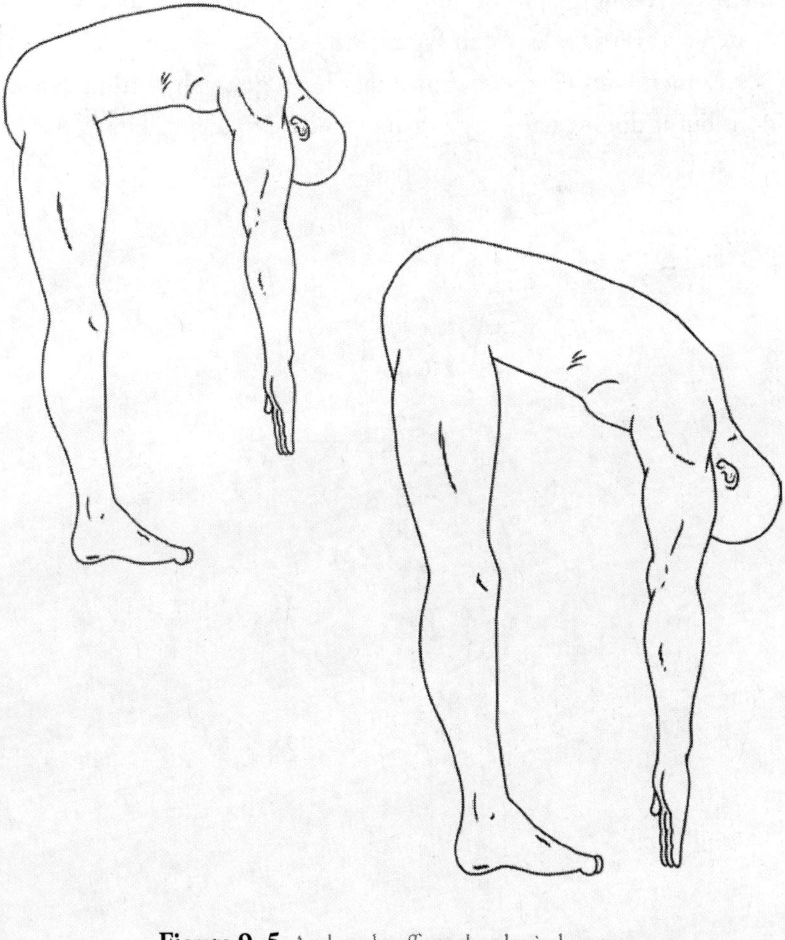

Figure 9. 5 As thought affects the physical posture

Tanden

Tanden is the physical and energetic center of our body. The most important center to maintain the body balanced. Hara is the abdomen area where the Tanden is located.

When we are in our natural state of balance, the tanden is located 3 or 4 cm below the navel. If we draw an imaginary line from the navel to the 3rd lumbar vertebra, and to the joints of the femur with the pelvic bones, we will find a triangle, the Tanden is located in the center of this triangle, see in Figure 9.6.

Tanden is an energetic center that has a great physical manifestation, but it doesn't have any organ or muscle to identify it.

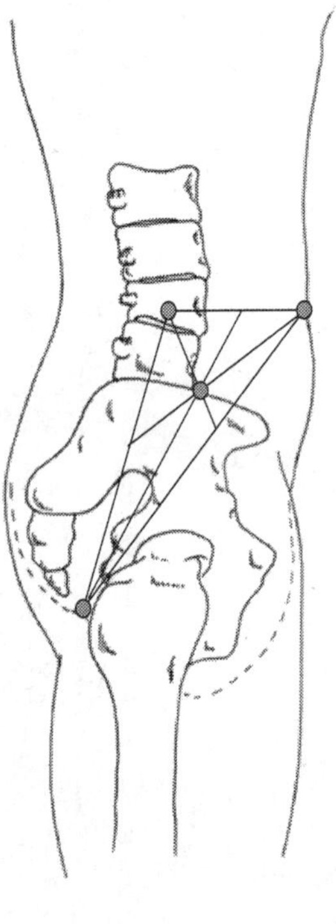

Figure 9. 6 Tanden

Localization of the Tanden

If for some reason we lose our natural state of balance, the Tanden's lacalization is modified.

For instance, when one leg is shorter than the other, due to a twisted pelvis, this body condition influences on the localization of theTanden, and on the whole physical and energetic balance of the body.

Our ancestors use to give great importance to this center. There are many roman sculptures of Jesus and of the roman virgins showing a prominent abdomen, as well as the ones of Buddha and Lao-Tsé in the East, symbolizing that they have a great Hara, meaning that they are centered in the Universe.

In all martial arts there are specific exercises to strengthen the Tanden. This happens because when a movement is made focused on Tanden, or when we use our force starting from the Tanden, we obtain much more power than when using only our muscular force.

On Samurais days, they trained their Tanden force, and used a Haramaki, a strip that was rolled up around the Hara, to strengthen the abdominal area.

In a Zen Buddhist meditations, called Zazen, They use to concentrate on the Tanden, to obtain a better physical and emotional balance.

The deep breathing also strengthens our Tanden.

When we are doing the deep breathing, expanding and emptying the abdomen, we strengthened our inner force. We develop a better physical, mental and emotional balance. The column is more erect, the thorax more expanded, the nervous system is more balanced and we improve our concentration capacity, as show in Figure 9.7.

In the traditional oriental medicine, Tanden and Hara are used to diagnose and to treat the body. Diagnosing on the Hara whether the energy is Kyo (empty) or Jitsu (full), then they look to reestablish the harmonic

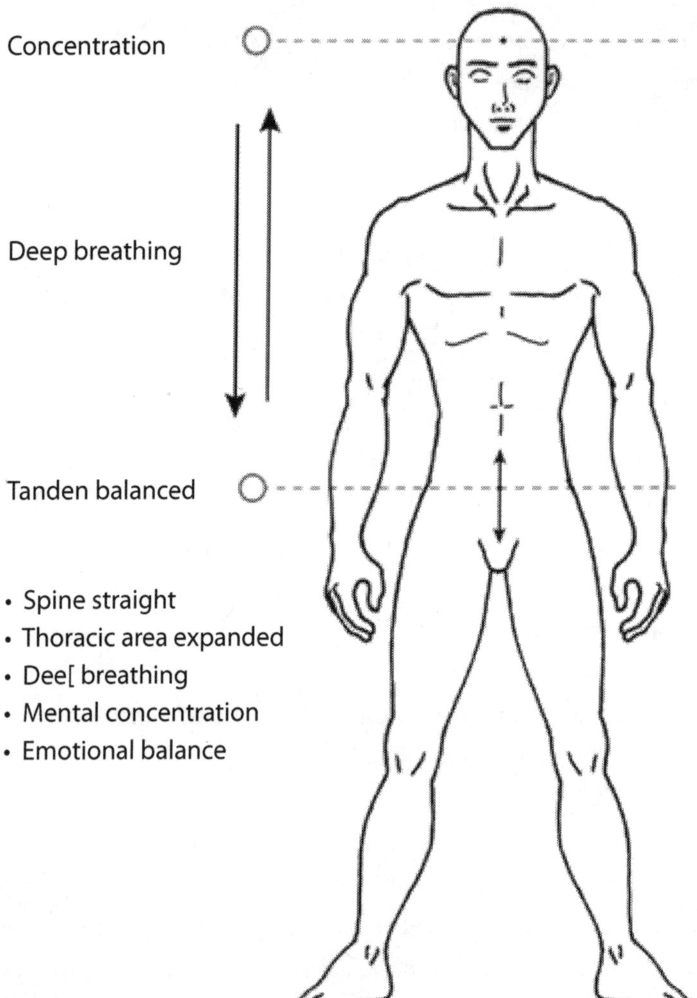

Figure 9. 7 Natural Posture develop Tanden and concentration

and balanced flow of Kyo and Jitsu. Through this balance, problems on other parts of the body can be cured. For instance, a lumbar pain may not mean a problem in the lumbar vertebrae, or in the muscular area of the lumbar region, but an unbalance in the Hara. Fallen organs could be causing this pain; by correcting the position of the internal organs we could cure that lumbar pain.

In the abdomen we have the representation of the whole body, as you can see in Figure 9.8. Depending where the pain in the abdomen is located, it indicates which related part of the body has a problem.

The upper part of the abdomen is related with the head and the mind. The central part is related with the organic part and the lumbar area. The low part of the abdomen is related with the legs.

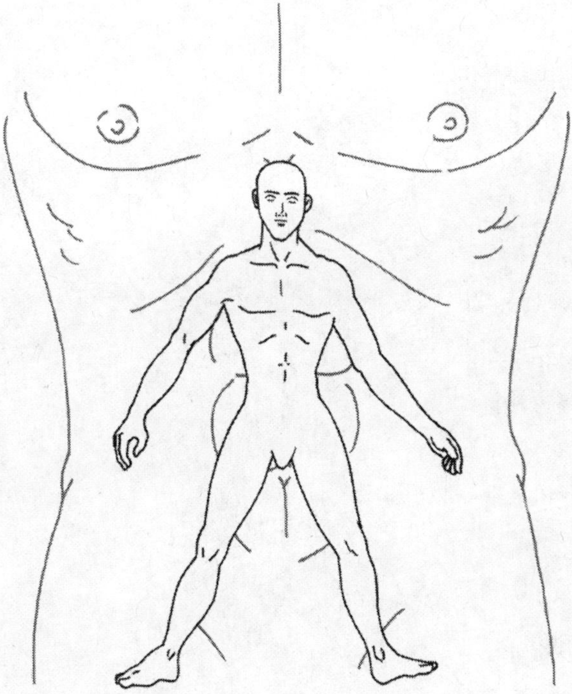

Figure 9. 8 The way of diagnosis in oriental medicine

We can compare the human body like a tree, as show in Figures 9,9 and 9.10. A good physical posture requires strong legs, and strength on the big toes to maintain a firm connection with the earth. The upper part of the body should be relaxed and flexible, with an open mind and good thoughts. We can say that this body is centered in its Tanden, in its own center.

On the other hand, if we don't have strong legs, and the upper part of our body becomes rigid, and we have a complicated and rigid mind, with tendency to neurosis, we won't be centered.

Vegetable kingdom

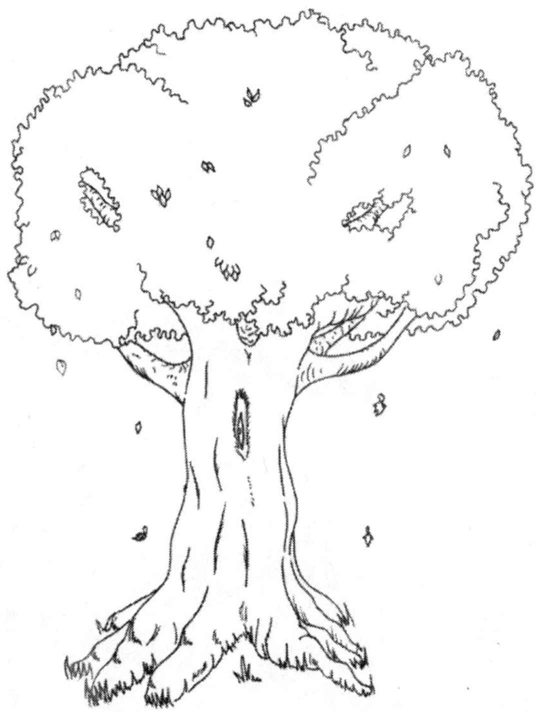

Figure 9. 9 Vegetable kingdom

When our legs are firm, it means that our organs are functioning well. When our legs are weakened, with circulatory problems, swollen, with varicose veins, this indicates that our organs are not functioning well. When our internal organs are fallen, extended, expanded, and the intestine are not functioning well, it disturbs the circulation of blood and vital energy through the legs.

When the body's upper part is more flexible and relaxed, we achieve a state of better emotional balance and clearer mind. But if the thoracic cage is closed, the chest and shoulders are contracted, we may have our

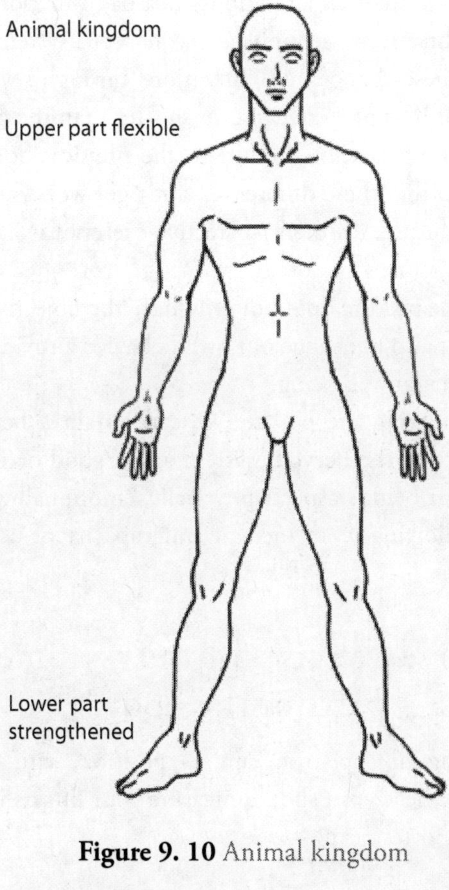

Figure 9. 10 Animal kingdom

emotional balance altered. Also we can have a tense nape and a neck without flexibility obstructing the blood flow to the head and brain, reducing our mental potentialities. Through exercises practice of strengthen the Tanden, we can corrected these alterations of the body, restoring our health condition and our physical, emotional and mental balance.

The body symmetry

When our body is on its natural condition, legs, arms, eyes, pelvic area, etc, are all symmetrical, in other words, they have the same size, they are equal.

When there are internal alterations, as a bad functioning of the organs, an altered breathing, an unbalanced nervous system, our physical body manifests these changes and alterations through several ways, like a misalignment of hips or spine, an arm shorter than the other. All these differences indicate a lack of balance in the physical body. They need to be corrected so that these differences don't get worse and cause more problems in the future. Through corrective exercises we can reestablish the balance and symmetry of the body.

Correcting the posture does not only have the objective to affect the physical body, but also to change our own behavior, providing a physical, emotional and mental well being.

Through correcting the posture we can obtain a better breathing condition, balance of the nervous system and a good organic functioning, improving our being's aspects physically, emotionally, mentally and also spiritually, allowing us to increase our capacity of using our inner potential.

Corrective exercise for the asymmetrical parts of the body

To diagnose: Lying face up - the "supine" position, with your arms extended above your head, you should measure your fingers joining length and identify the shortest arm.

The shortening of the arm indicates a blockade of the internal energy on this arm. The lung on this same side can be more contracted; the nostril on this side can be more closed than the other, indicating that the breathing on this side doesn't flow as much as on the opposite side.

Treating: to correct the arms length, press a point on the internal corner of the eye, see in Figure 9.11, at the beginning of the eyebrow, on the same side of the shortest arm. Massage this point for about 3 minutes, until it relieves.

To check: after having pressed the point, extend again your arms above your head and check the length of the arms. They should be the same length or almost the same.

- How to check
- The point to be pressed.

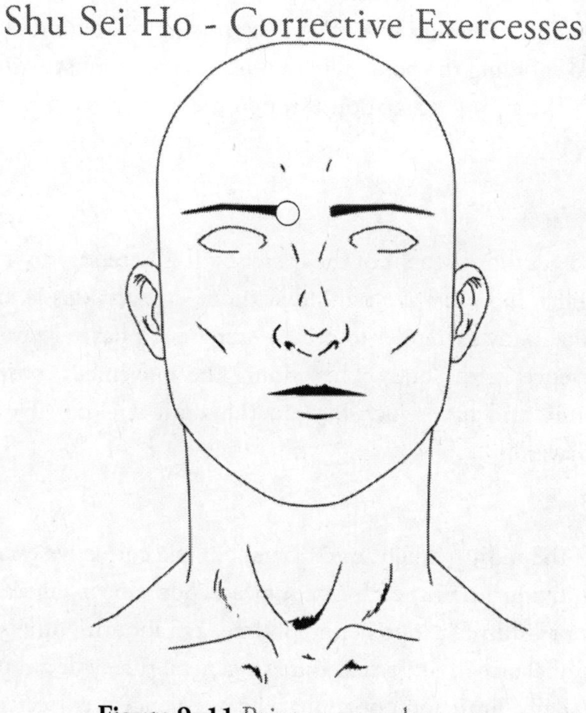

Figure 9. 11 Point to treat short arm

Basic notions for practicing the corrective exercises

Physical posture:

- Do all exercises concentrating on Tanden.
- Relax the shoulders, so that you don't tension it when doing the exercise, when you are making the effort.
- If the exercise is done with the person seated or lying down, he/she should always keep the Aquilis tendon stretched, so that the toes stay upward, strengthen like this the Tanden.
- On the standing exercises, transfer your body weight to your big toe.

Breathing:

Inhale through the nose, expanding the abdomen.

Exhale through the mouth whenever you do the physical effort of the movement. This way you will be increasing the elimination of the toxins, and avoiding the possibility of tensioning the musculature due to the effort. The strong exhalation through the mouth let the body more alkaline.

Mental attitude:

- To get more benefit of the exercises, it is necessary to unite body and mind. To have a mind without expectations is ideal for a total body surrender to do the exercise. To have always the conscience in the body when doing the movement, observing its limit, and haw much beyond this limit it is possible to move forward.

Quantity:

This is the most frequent question about the corrective exercis-es. It is a very individual point, each case is a case. Some people need to practice a lot more, during a long period of time, as 3 months, others can correct their unbalance in one week. But as a general rule, you can practice 5 to 8 times, daily, until you notice that the unbalance is corrected.

Relaxation:

After practicing the corrective exercise, it is necessary some minutes of relaxation for the body to assimilate the changes. The relaxation should be made lying on a supine position -face up, with the arms placed along the body, and the palms of the hands facing up, the maxillary relaxed, and the tongue placed in the roof of the mouth, see Figure 9.12. Stay in this position approximately 3 minutes, with a natural and deep breathing.

Relaxation posture

- lying on the ground with the belly upward.

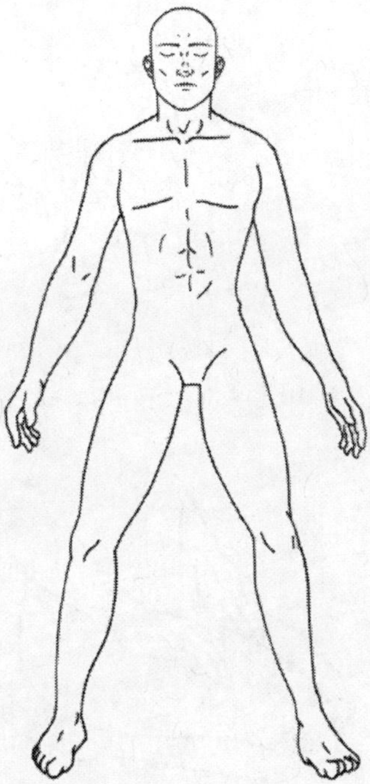

Figure 9.12 Relaxation Posture

Seiza posture

This posture is very common in Japan, it is used in several situations, such as watching TV, reading, during the meals, drinking tea, and meditating.

This posture strengthens the Tanden and the whole lower part of the body, allowing the expansion of thoracic cage and as a consequence a deeper breathing, see Figure 9.13.

They seat in seiza during the meals, so that the stomach is not pressed by any of the internal organs or ribs. And they also seat in seiza to meditate, because this posture let the spine straight and stimulates concentration and conscience expansion.

Posture: seating on the ground, with your legs flexed, knees two fists width. The pelvic area placed in between the heels, big toes on top of each other. The spine straight, shouders relaxed, chest expanded, the nape of the neck prolonged and the chin in, see in Figure 9.13.

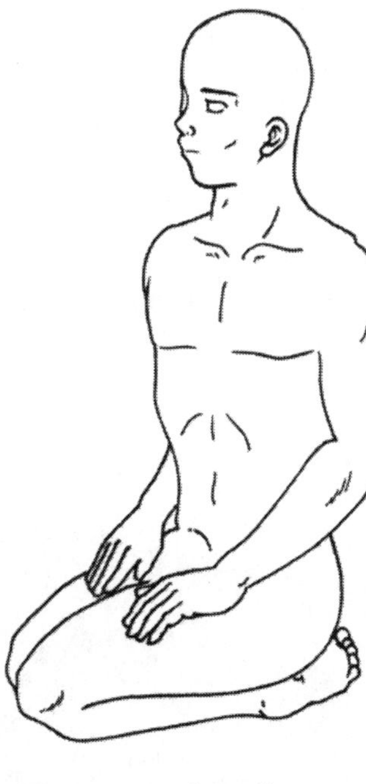

Figura 9.13 Seiza Posture

Fish Posture:

This posture will be used for many of the following corrective exercises.

It brings by itself several benefits to the organism, such as: expands the thorax, allowing a deep breath, relieves the tensions in the shoulders and strengthens the physical center of the body.

Posture: lying on your back, place the elbows on the ground beside the chest, with the fists closed. Rest the head's top on the floor, stretch out the legs and the Achilles tendons, as show in Figure 9.14.

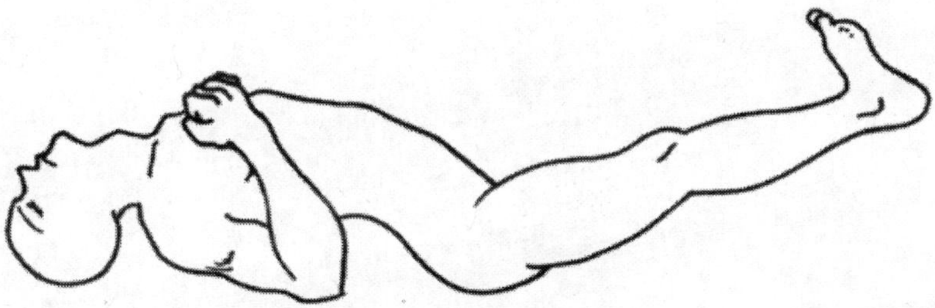

Figure 9 . 14 Fish Posture

10

Tanden

Exercises to strengthen the Tanden

1 – posture: two people, seating in seiza, one in front of the other. One seats with his/her knees open, and the other with his/her knees in the space between the former knees, see in Figure 10.1.

Motion: Inhale and when exhaling, the person that is with the knees inside tries to open his/her legs, forcing open the partner's legs.

Both should breath synchronized.

This movement strengthens the whole pelvic area musculature, and brings power to Tanden.

2 – posture: two people, one standing and the other lying down, with his/her legs stretched upward making a 90º degree angle with the floor, holding the ankle of standing up person, keeps the elbows and arms touching the floor, and the Achilles tendon stretched, see in Figure 10.2.

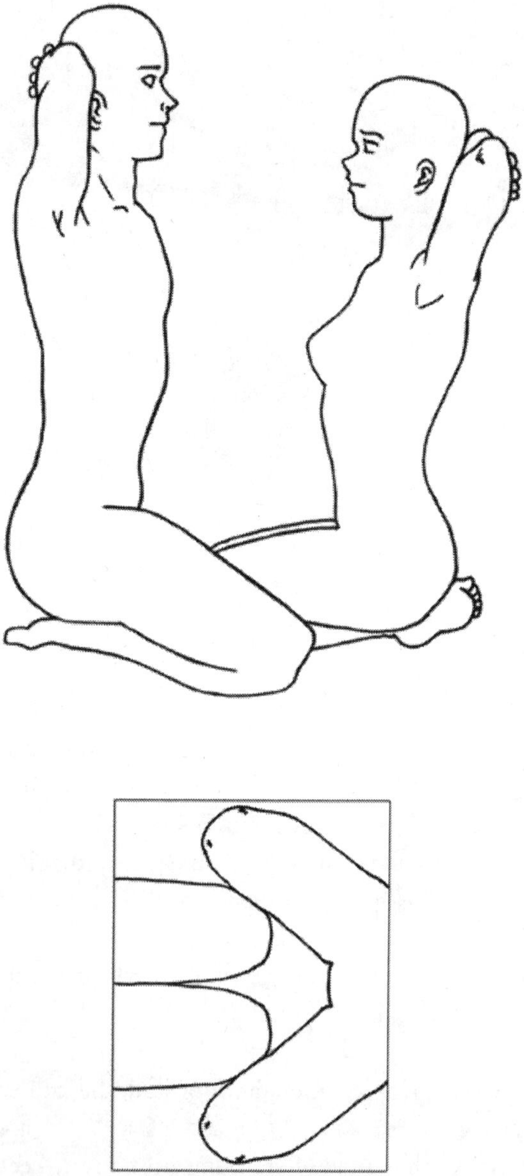

Figure 10. 1 Exercise nº 1 to strengthen the tanden

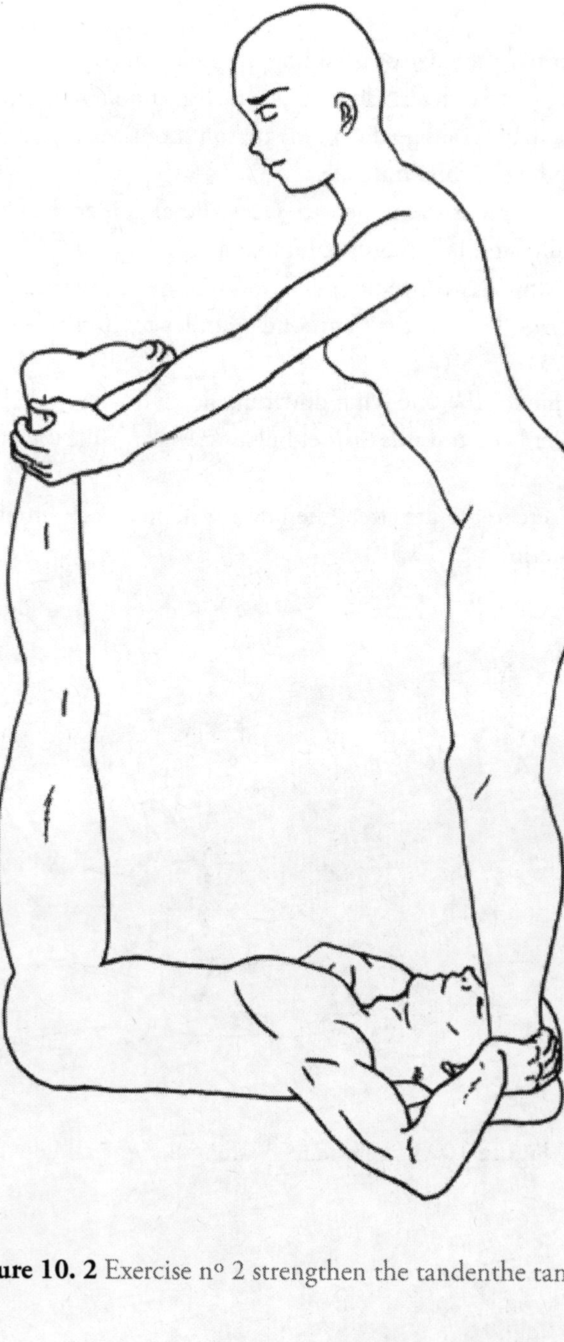

Figure 10. 2 Exercise n° 2 strengthen the tandenthe tanden

Movement: the person standing up, holds the other one ankle, and pushes them into different directions. The legs should not touch the floor. Every time his/her legs go down, the person should exhale and every time they go up he/she should inhale.

This movement strengthens the legs and abdomen area, it improves legs flexibility and it loosens the lumbar area.

3 – posture: two people, one lying face down, with the chin leaning on his/her hands, legs bent, and Achilles tendon stretched, see in Figure 10.3.

Movement: The one lying down inhale, and when exhaling tries to bring his/her heels towards his/her buttocks, meanwhile the other person makes resistance.

This exercise besides strengthening the Tanden, also strengthens the thigh's posterior muscles.

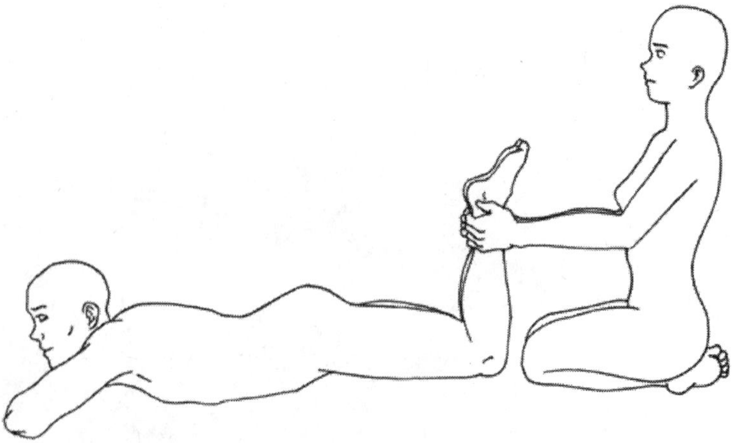

Figure 10. 3 Exercise nº 3 strengthen the tanden

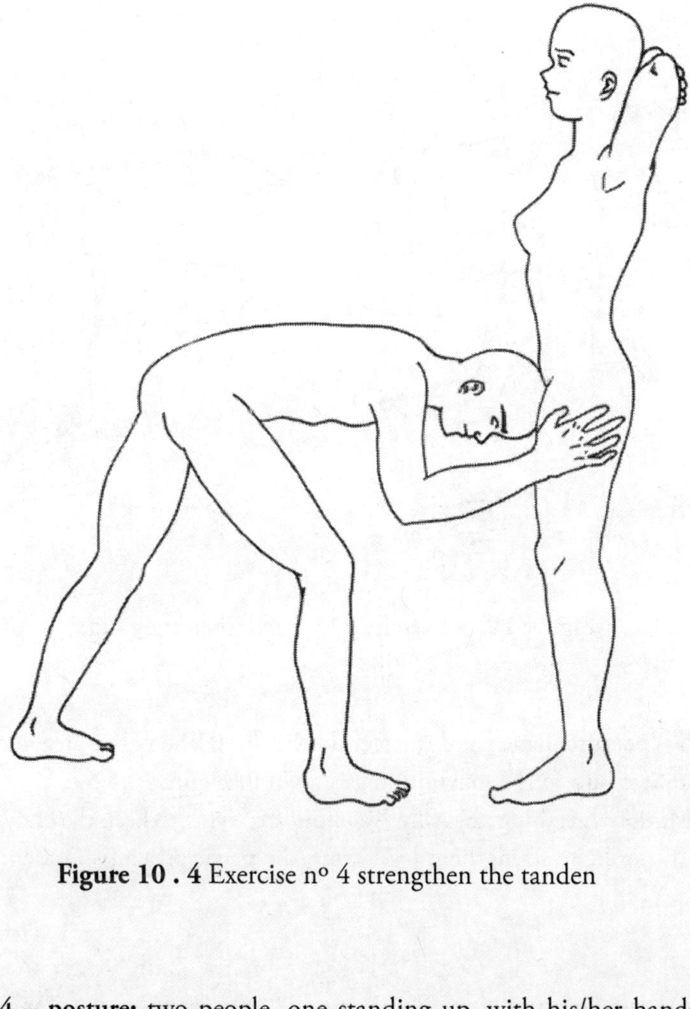

Figure 10 . 4 Exercise nº 4 strengthen the tanden

4 – posture: two people, one standing up, with his/her hands interlaced behind his/her head, the other with his/her head leaning on the partner's tanden and the hands on his/her hips′ bones, see in Figure 10.4.

Movement: the person standing up, tries to move forward, exhaling at each step and bringing all his/her power to his/her Hara. The other resists using his/her head and hands, but allows the person to move with a certain difficulty.

This exercise strengthens Tanden and legs.

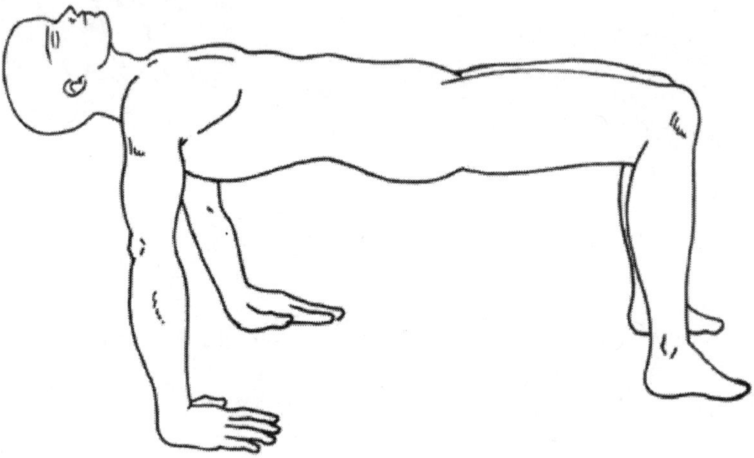

Figure 10. 5 Exercise nº 5 strengthen the tanden

5 – **posture:** hands and the feet on the floor. The pelvic area and the trunk, lifted up to the maximum, as shown in Figure 10.5.

Motion: breathing normally, walk forward trying to keep the body up.

This exercise strengthens legs, arms, the pelvic area and Tanden.

Kiai

It is a shout, commonly used in the martial arts, to strengthen Tanden.

Actually it is a breathing exercise. You inhale deeply and when exhaling shout "Kiai", the sound should come from the abdomen. It's a good exercise to take away fear, relaxes shoulders and the mind, and strengthens the low part of the abdomen.

Kiai exercises to strengthen the Tanden.

1 – posture: individual exercise. Stand up, with feet parallel, distant hips width, as show in Figure 10.6.

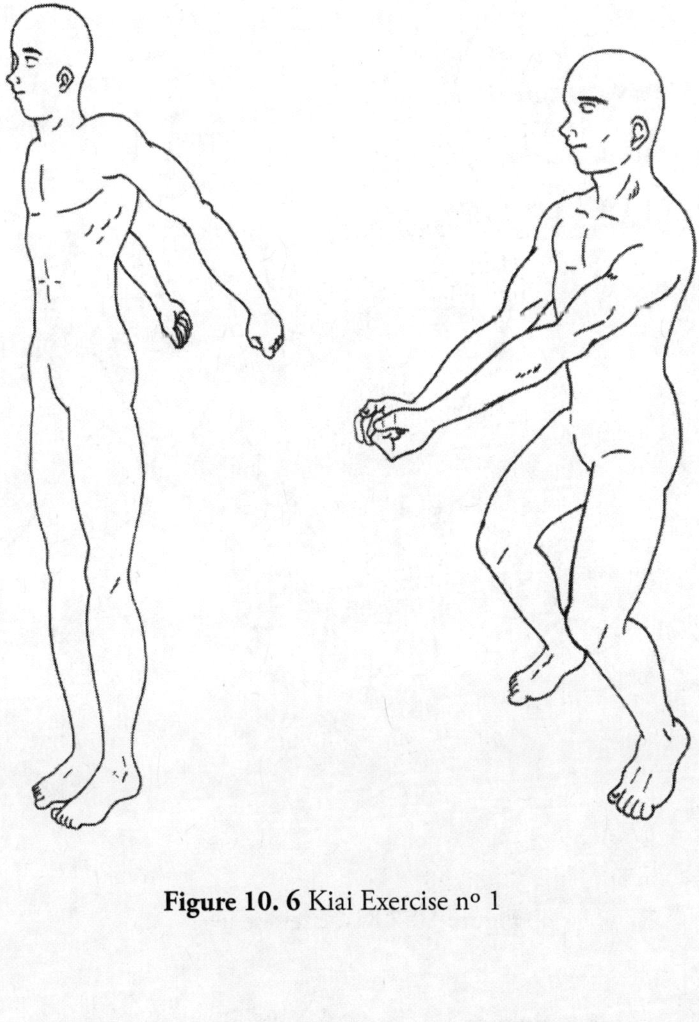

Figure 10. 6 Kiai Exercise nº 1

Motion: inhaling bring your arms back with fist closed and thumbs in. Raise your heels and stand on your tip toes.

Exhaling shout Kiai, bring your heels down, and landing your feet on the floor, inflecting the knees a little and lifting the arms parallel ahead your body. Keeping your spine straight and anus closed.

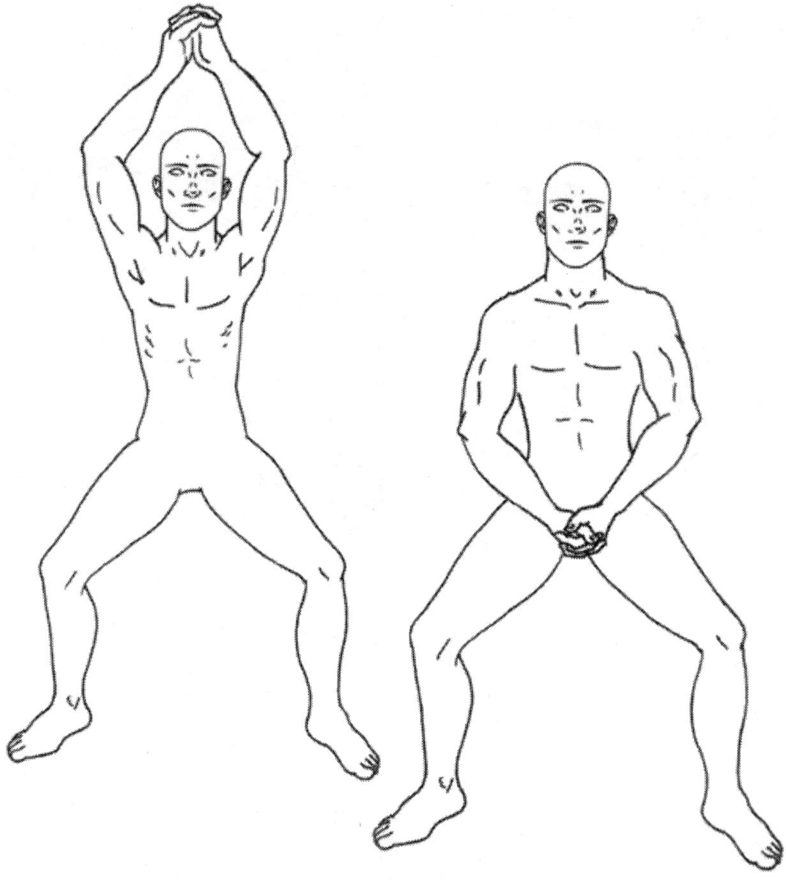

Figure 10.7 Kiai Exercise nº 2

2 – posture: Stand up, legs apart, feet slightly open, keep your spine straight during the exercise.

Motion: When inhaling bring your arms upward, with your fingers interlaced and knees bent, and exhaling bring your arms down vigorously, touching the abdomen and letting out the Kiai shout, as show in Figure 10.7.

Keep your buttocks and the abdomen contracted.

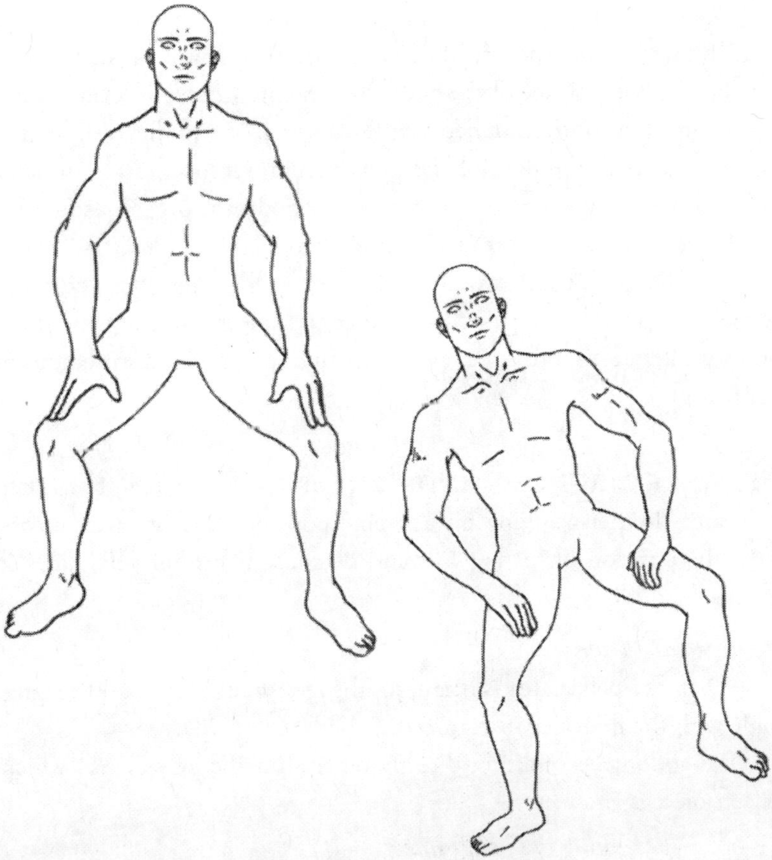

Figure 10. 8 Kiai Exercise nº 3

3 – posture: standing, with your legs inflected and apart. Feet slightly looking out, and with your hands leaning on your knees, see in Figure 10.8.

Motion: inhaling lift up one of your legs of the floor, and exhaling bring this leg down beating your foot on the floor, and letting out the kiai shout.

Repeat the same movement with the other leg.

Koshi Pelvic area

The pelvic area (pelvis, hips, sacral bone) is of a great importance for the physical balance of the body, because the Tanden is located in its center. It is the connection between the upper part and the lower part of our body. It is also responsible for great part of our locomotion. It holds and it protects a very important part of our body, the organs responsible for the perpetuation of our species, our reproductive organs.

When our body feels any alteration in the pelvic area, it can be manifested as lumbar pains, pains in the legs and knees, poor organic functioning, alterations in the genital organs, and for women disturbances in her period.

How to diagnose unbalances in the pelvic area

With the person lying on a supine position, face up, we can observe the position of his/her feet and diagnose if his/her pelvic area is balanced.

Balanced way.

When the pelvic area is balanced, the feet should form a 60° degree angle with the floor, see in Figure 10.9.

The abdomen condition directly reflects on the pelvic area, which reflects on legs and feet.

a – Hips leaning to the left side

When the left leg is more fallen, as show in Figure 10.10, and we notice that the left foot has a very small angle with the floor, it indicates that the left side of the abdomen is empty (kyo), flaccid, possibly with the organs fallen to this side.

While the abdomen on the right side is contracted, stiffened, and the organs on this side overloaded, the kidneys and the liver with excess of energy.

The person frequently fells pain or discomfort on the right side of the body. They can be muscular pain, stiff neck, pain of the sciatic nerve, or lumbar pain, all on the right side.

This condition is more common in people that have a more practical attitude before life.

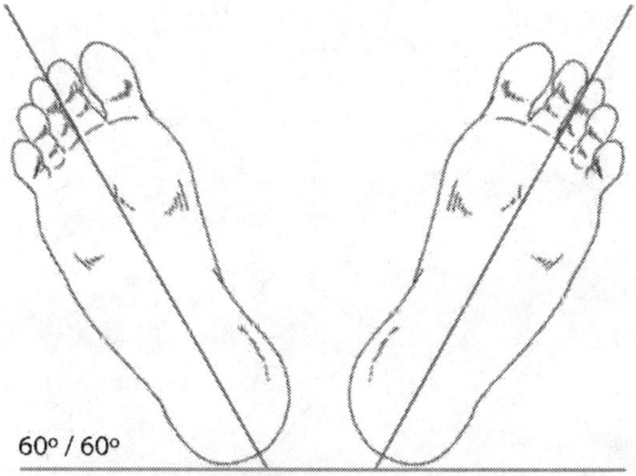

Figure 10.9 Balanced feet

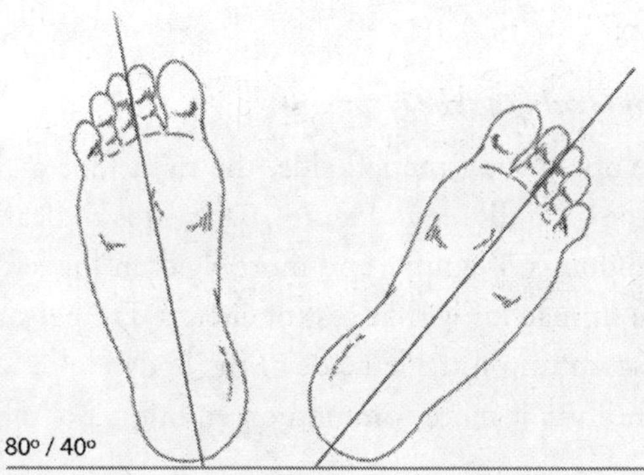

Figure 10.10 pelvis twisted to the right

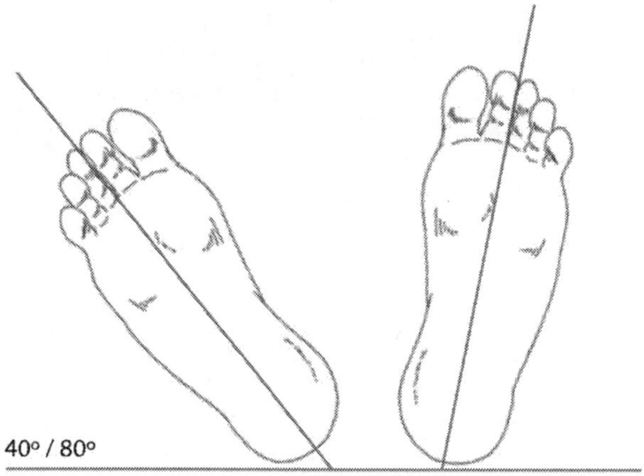

Figure 10. 11 pelvis twisted to the left

b – Hips leaning to the right side

It is the opposite of the left side, the right foot makes a very small angle with the ground, see in Figure 10.11. This indicates that the right side of the abdomen is empty, and more rigid on the left side.

And the stomach is with excess of energy. The person frequently has a pain or discomfort on the left side of the body.

This condition is more common on emotional or creative people.

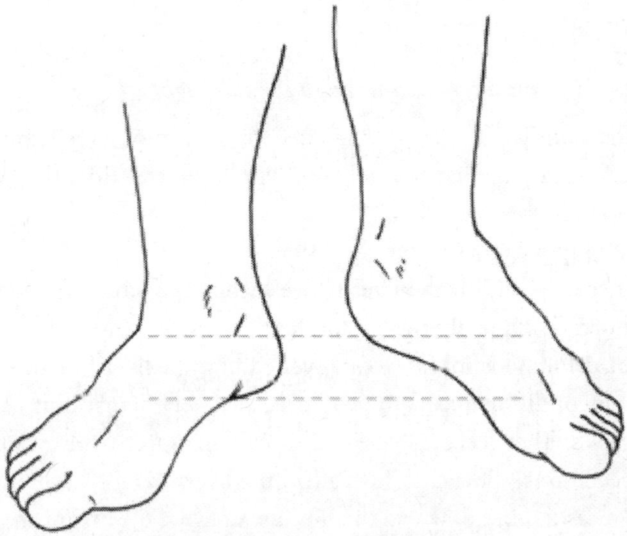

Figure 10.12 Short left leg

c – Hips misaligned, uneven to the left side

The left leg is shorter than the right leg. Comparing the heels, we can see that the left leg is shorter than the right leg, as show in Figure 10.12.

The hip bone is higher on the left side.

It indicates that the stomach is overloaded, could be with an ulcer or gastritis. This condition of the organ makes the right side of the abdomen to contract, causing an upward unevenness of the hip bane.

In general, when the person had very demanding parents, that passed to him/her as a child a lot of tension, making him/her worried and nervous, these feelings can affect the stomach functions.

d – Hips misaligned, uneven to the side right

The right leg is shorter than the left, we can observe this looking at the persons' heels, that the right leg will be shorter than the left , see in Figure 10.13.

The hip is higher to the right side.

In this condition the liver is overloaded, possibly expanded, bigger than normal. Probably the person has a rich diet, eats too much greasy food or drinks alcohol in excess, overloading the liver functions. In general, this condition occurs to people that are very demanding or critics to themselves. They feel anger because they don't meet their own demands, or expectations, these emotions affect the liver.

On cases c and d, where the hips are uneven, the organism presents a very favorable condition to create a scoliosis. The bad functioning of the internal organs, liver and stomach, plus the twist of the pelvic area, favors an unbalance, a misalignment of the spine. We notice that the corrective exercises for the pelvic bones, hips, are essential to prevent possible problems on the spine.

When a person has scoliosis, it is necessary to correct the internal organs first, afterwards the pelvic bones, and then to align the spine with stretching and corrective exercises.

In the case of a leg shorter than the other, usually people choose to put an inner sole in their shoe, on the shortest leg side. However we don't recommend the use of the inner sole, because it doesn't correct the twisted hips, and it takes our possibility to correct our body. Through corrective exercises we can correct and find balance to great majority of the cases. The inner sole is only advisable for cases that one side of the bones become shorter due to bad congenital formation, accident or surgery.

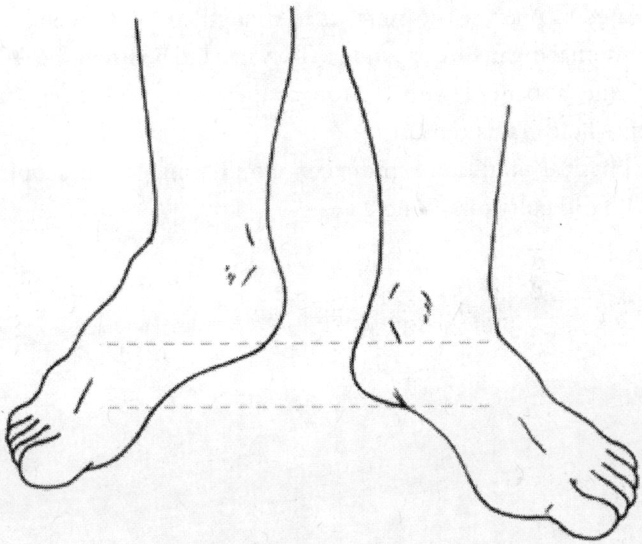

Figure 10.13 Short right leg

e – Pelvic bones too open, fallen feet.

When the feet fall totally to the sides, it indicates that the pelvic bones are very closed on the back and very opened on the front, and the iliac bones are apart, as show in Figure 10.14.

It also indicates that the Tanden is very weak, he/she some how is losing his/her vital force, or is not using his/her body appropriately.

In this case, besides the corrective exercises for the pelvic bones, hips, it is indicated to practice the exercises to strengthen the Tanden.

The internal organs are expanded. They need to be strengthened with exercises, and also need with a stronger diet, with vegetables, cooked roots, and whole grains cereals.

This physical condition is more common on undecided people, and people with difficulty to say "no".

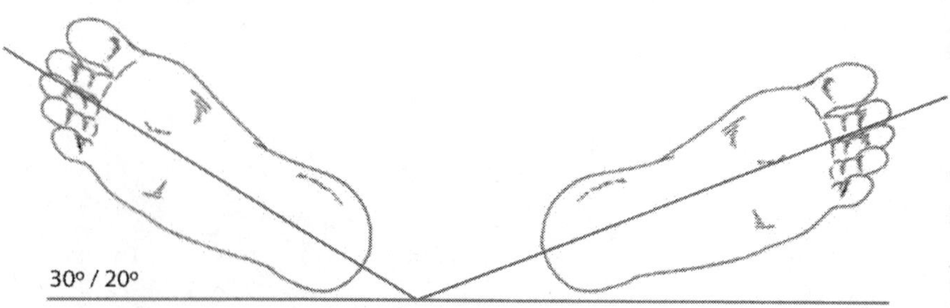

Figure 10.14 Open pelvic bone

f – contracted pelvic area (hips), closed feet .

When the feet are with the big toes closed in, and heels open, it indicates that there are a lot of tension and rigidity in the internal organs. This tension contracts the abdomen, closing like this the iliac bones, as show in Figure 10.15.

In general, this physical condition is common on people that have a lot of internal conflicts. People with difficulty to express themselves or that have an introverted and closed behavior.

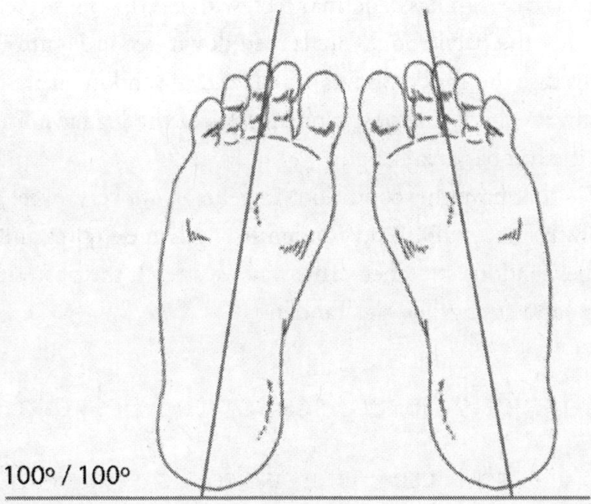

Figure 10. 15 Pelvis closed

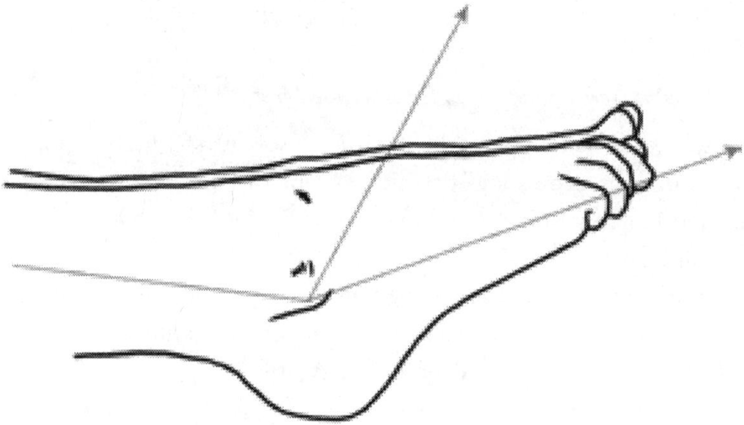

Figure 10. 16 Posture of the feet in the shy person

g – Pelvic bones leaned down, with the tip toes downward.

When the person has ballerina's feet, with the tip toes stretched down, it means that the pelvic bones are leaned down, see in Figure 10.16.

In this case the Tanden is weakened, and the abdomen area below the navel is always rigid. The posterior muscles of the leg have little stretching, and the lumbar area is tight.

People that have this condition, in general, are very sweet and shy.

It's always necessary to do Tanden strengthen exercises and maintain the Achilles tendons stretched. This way we stretch the posterior muscles of our legs and strengthen the Tanden.

Corrective exercises for the pelvic area

1 – corrective exercise for case a or b:

To diagnose: With the person lying down, in a relaxation posture, verify which foot is fallen more to the side.

Posture: The person lying down, with his/her Achilles tendons stretched. The other seated holds the person's feet.

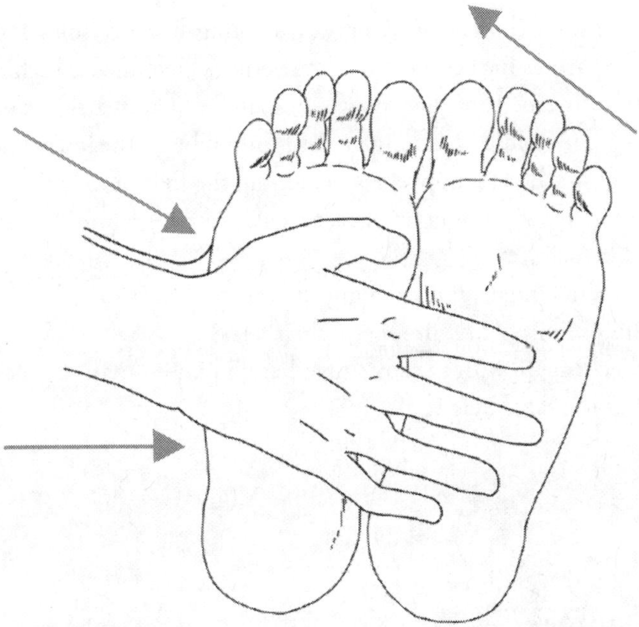

Fig**ure 10.17** Corrective exercise case B

Motion: If the foot on the right side is fallen more, the person that is lying down inhale and exhaling pushes his/her feet to the right side. The other person, using his/her hands, resists to that force, see in Figure 10.17.

Both should breathe together.

If it is the left foot the more fallen one, you should do the same movement, but pushing to the left side.

Repeat this exercise 5 to 8 times and then relax.

To check: in the relaxation posture, check if the leg that was more fallen is no balanced in relation to the other leg. If they are still not on the same height, repeat the exercise.

2 – corrective exercise for cases a or b:

To diagnose: the person lying down, bring his/ her soles together and knees apart, as in the drawing, then verify which knee is higher.

Posture: the person lying down, put his/her hands behind his/her head, knees bent and feet leaning on the ground, bring the lower knee towards the ground, to its opposite side, letting the foot out. At the higher knee side his/her leg should be perpendicular to the ground , see in Figure 10.18.

Movement: inhale and exhaling lift up the hips to the maximum. Repeat this exercise 5 to 8 times and then relax.

To check: again with the soles together and knees apart, check if the knees are at the same height.

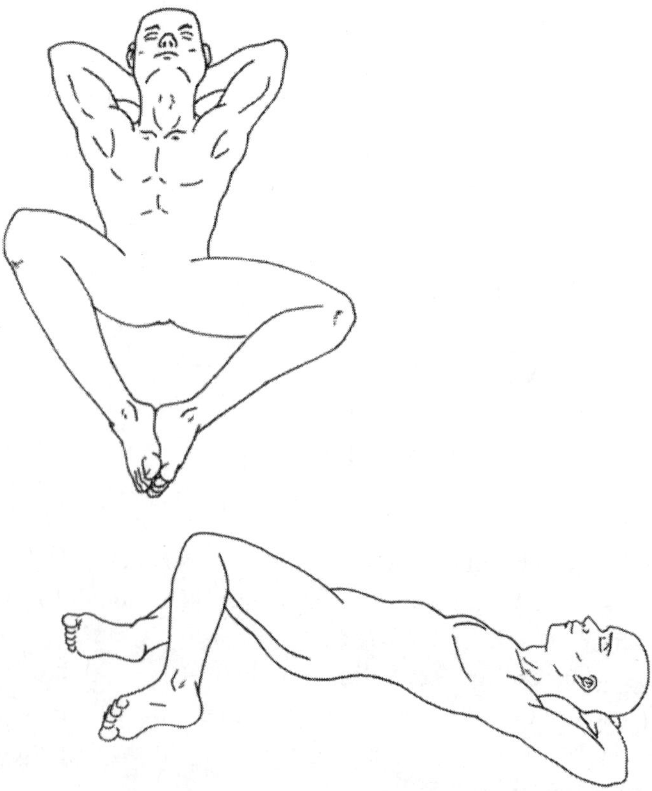

Figure 10.18 Corretive exercise case B

3 – corrective exercise for cases a or b:

To diagnose: with the person lying, face up, on the relaxation posture, check which foot is fallen more to the side.

Posture: the person lying down, bend his/her knees, feet sole leaning on the ground, place the fallen foot close to his/her hips and the other far from the hips.

Movement: In the relaxation posture inhale, and exhaling lift up the hips. Repeat this exercise 5 to 8 times and then relax, as show in Figure 10.19.

To check: in the relaxation posture, check if the feet are equal, at the same height.

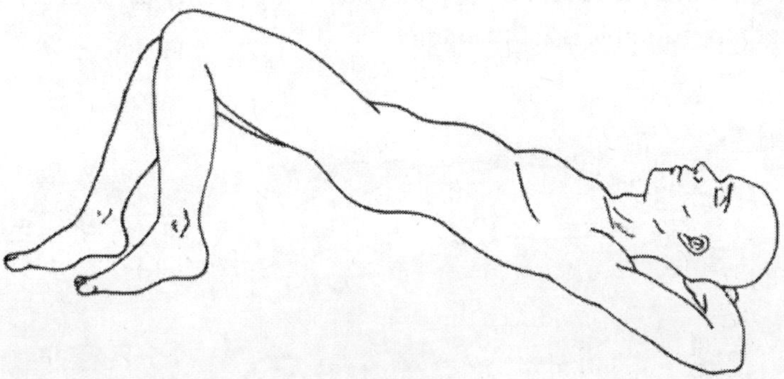

Figure 10.19 Corretive exercise case B

4 – Corrective exercise for cases c and d:

To diagnose: lying on the relaxation posture, verify which leg is shorter than the other. You can see the difference comparing the two heels, seen if one is shorter than the other.

Posture: the person lying down, arms stretched above his/her head, shorter leg extended on the ground, the Achilles tendon stretched, and the longer leg bent open to the side, and knee close to ground, see in Figure 10.20.

Motion: the person lying down Inhale, and when exhaling lift his/her body up bringing his/her hands towards the foot, trying to touch it. If necessary, the partner can hold the person's ankle of his/her extended leg, supporting him/her to lift up his/her body.

Repeat this exercise 5 to 8 times and then to relax.

To check: in the relaxation posture, observing his/her heels, check if the length of his/her legs are the same.

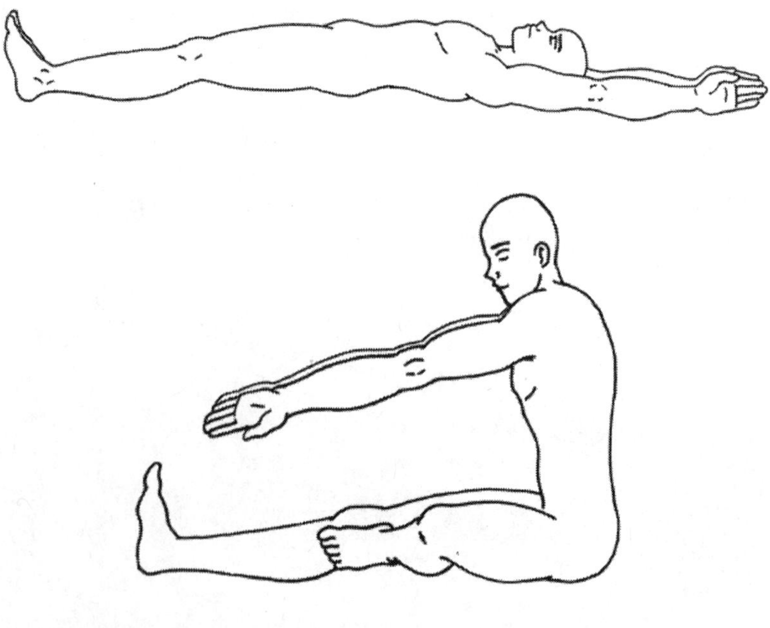

Figure 10.20 Corretive exercise case D

5 – Corrective exercise for case e:

To diagnose: the person lying on the relaxation posture, verify if his/her feet are fallen too much to the sides, with the tips bending sideways, almost touching the floor.

Posture: the person lying, his/her knees bent backwards with his/her feet beside the thighs, and arms extended above the head, see in Figure 10.21.

Movement: The person inhale and exhaling lift up his /her trunk, keeping his /her arms stretched. If necessary, the partner can hold the person's knees, giving him/her support to accomplish the movement.

Repeat the exercise 5 to 8 times and then relax.

To check: on the relaxation posture, check if his/her feet are more closed, and if the angle between the feet and the ground is closer to 60º.

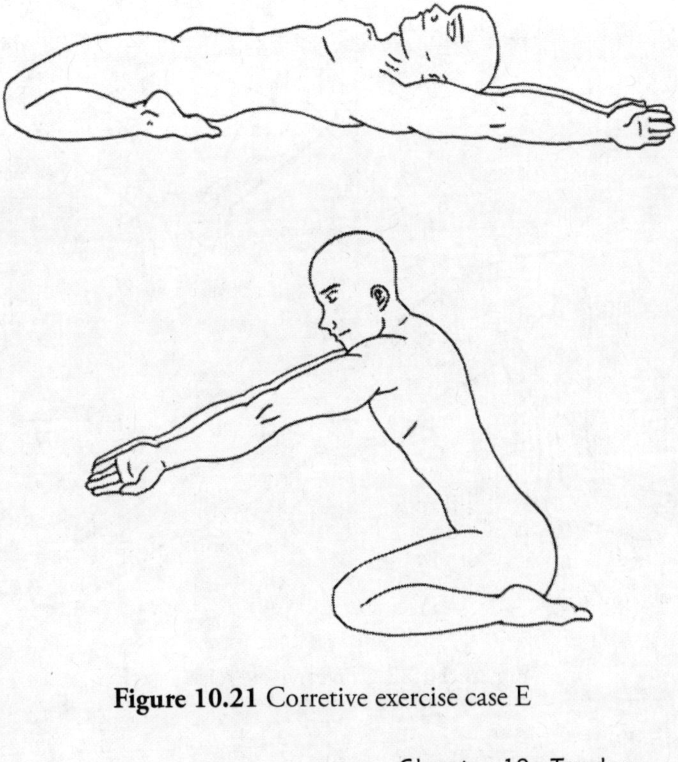

Figure 10.21 Corretive exercise case E

6 – Corrective exercise for case f:

To diagnose: the person lying down on the relaxation posture, the partner verifies if his/her feet are facing in, closed.

Posture: the person lying down, hands behind the nape of his/her neck, soles together, knees bend and open, see in Figure 10.22.

Movement: The person lying down inhale and when exhaling lift his/her hips up to the maximum, opening the front side of his/her pelvic area and closing the back side.

Repeat this exercise 5 to 8 times and then to relax.

To check: the person lies on the relaxation posture, and the partner check if his/her feet are more open.

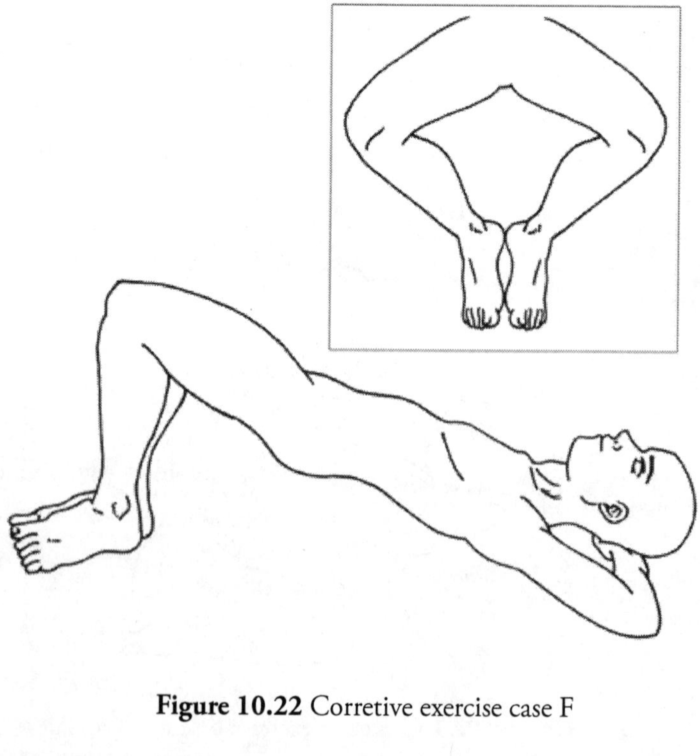

Figure 10.22 Corretive exercise case F

7 – Corrective exercise for case g:

To diagnose: the person lying on the relaxation posture, the partner verifies if his/her tip toes are facing down, as a ballerinas' feet.

Posture: the person lying down, stretches his/ her arms above his/her head, with his/her hands' palms turned out, legs extended and the Achilles tendons stretched.

Movement: the person inhale, and exhaling lift his/her trunk up, bringing his/her hands towards his/her feet. If necessary, the partner can hold the person's ankles, giving him /her support to accomplish the movement, as show in Figure 10.23.

Repeat this exercise 5 to 8 times and then relax.

To check: the person lying down on the relaxation posture, check if his/her toes are looking more vertical.

In this case, the person should practice this series once a day, for many days, until his/her pelvic area (hips) is balanced again.

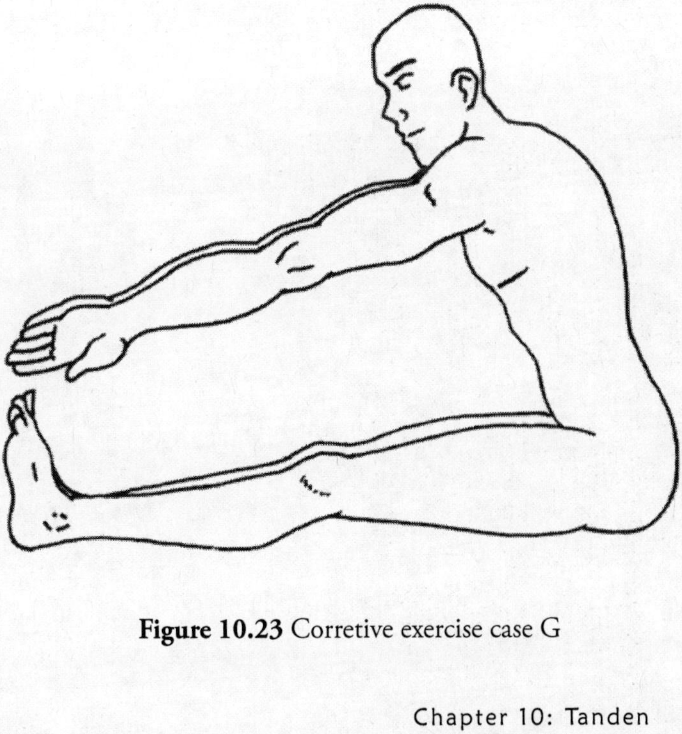

Figure 10.23 Corretive exercise case G

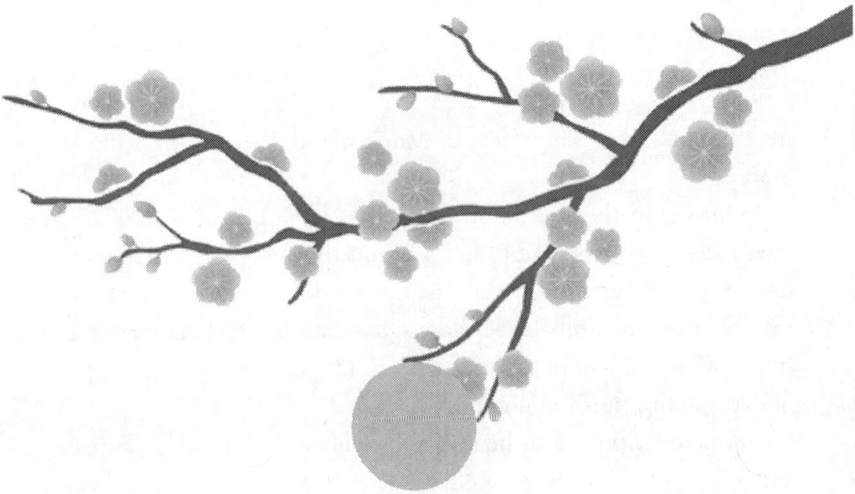

Conclusions of the authors

Author's note

I had the opportunity to meet Masahiro Oki when he came to Rio deJaneiro in 1982. He invited me to go to Japan to learn and train his teachings and, later, to disclose them in South America. In January 1983, I went to New York, where I lived in the dojo of Koji Yamamoto, who was already a student of Oki sensei and disclosed his teachings in the United States. There, I perfected my English and began my training in these techniques. From there I went to Mishima, to the dojo of Oki sensei, where I lived for two years. Oki sensei's training was very strict; we would wake up at 5:30 am and we would have intense activities throughout the day, up to 10:00 pm. This period of my life was very outstanding; I learned micchio, which is the teaching passed on practically and not only intellectually.

After returning from Japan, where I accompanied the treatment of Masahiro Oki of various physical and psychic alterations, I began my works in Laranjeiras, in Rio de Janeiro, in 1984. I gradually began to minister courses and built a clientele in various parts of Brazil, like Rio de Janeiro, Espírito Santo, Santa Catarina, São Paulo and Mato Grosso. As time went by, I extended my work to other countries, in several places in Argentina, in Cuernavaca, in Mexico, and New York, in the United States.

During all these years of experience, having treated over 20 thousand cases of various symptoms and pains through the Oki-Do method, I have obtained very positive effects. I noticed that migraines or headaches treated as organic imbalance had a significant improvement after 10 sessions. With a higher number of sessions (approximately 20), the pictures of depression improved notably.

Kanrenbui proved to be a very beneficial technique for human balance.

Treatment should be done not through symptoms, but through strengthening of the tanden, the physical and energy center of the body, leading the person to develop better harmony of the body and mind. It is therefore a more holistic treatment.

With a dedicated and conscious practice, one can provide a therapy without side effects and with excellent results to several people with some type of imbalance or health deficiency.

— *Fernando Montoto*

Author's note

Once, in the Orient, a man went to meet a sufi master, seeking to be accepted by him as a disciple and to receive his teachings. He waited for several days until he was received by the master. On arriving in his presence, he said: "Master, I came to seek your teachings". The master did not answer and asked another disciple to bring them tea. On filling his teacup, the master did not stop pouring the tea from the pot. The cup overflowed and the tea was already spreading on the tray when the man said quickly: "Master, the tea is spilling…". The master, finally, spoke to him, saying. "Like your mind, this

cup is full and there is no space for more tea. Go and empty your mind, only them come back to learn".

Since 1986, when I have been to Japan to learn and live in the *dojo* of Oki sensei, I have used these teachings daily in my life and in my clinic.

When I write a book passing on the teachings I received in Japan and the great learning of my intensive clinical experience, I feel my body emptying. Thus, I have space for the new.

For me, knowledge passed on is living; knowledge kept is dead!

Therefore, on reading this book, first empty yourself of your attachments to the knowledge you already have. *Kanrenbui* is a method whose characteristic is the simplicity of the Orient and a conception of the body completely different from that of the Occident. Secondly, leave it in a place where you can easily take it: in your room, table or office. Do not keep it in the drawer or shelf. Use it, apply these points on yourself. Press your foot or your hand while you watch TV or browse the internet. Press the points in your family, friends, clients or patients. This way, this knowledge will be alive in your life, as it is in mine.

— *Paula Guimarães*

Paula Guimarães is Brazilian, born in 1963. She started to study and practice the natural food, shiatsu and yoga when she was 20 years old. She travelled to Japan at 22 years old to deepen her knowledge on oriental medicine, there graduating from Masahiro Oki School called Oki Yoga Dojo, in the city of Mishima. Returning to Brazil, she opened her oriental therapy center and school, which has professional courses on shiatsu, the Okido Terapia Corporal in São Paulo.

Fernando Montoto trained and lived with Masahiro Oki in Mishima in Japan during the years 1983 and 1984, becoming part of the staff and making public the oriental medicine techniques in the Latin America countries.

Currently he teaches and consultation services in São Paulo (where he lives), Cuiabá and Santa Catarina.

Paula Guimarães and Fernando Montoto disclose their experiences in progress and techniques in Brazil and also in Argentina, Mexico, United States and Japan.

Authors Publishing:

- Relações do corpo [Body relations];
- Shusei Ho, manual de exercícios corretivos [corrective exercises handbook]
- Shiatsu Volume 1 – Book + DVD

Bibliographic Reference

PUTZ, R., PABST, R., Atlas de Anatomia Humana Sobotta. 22nd Edition, Editora Guanabara Koogan, Rio de Janeiro, 2006.

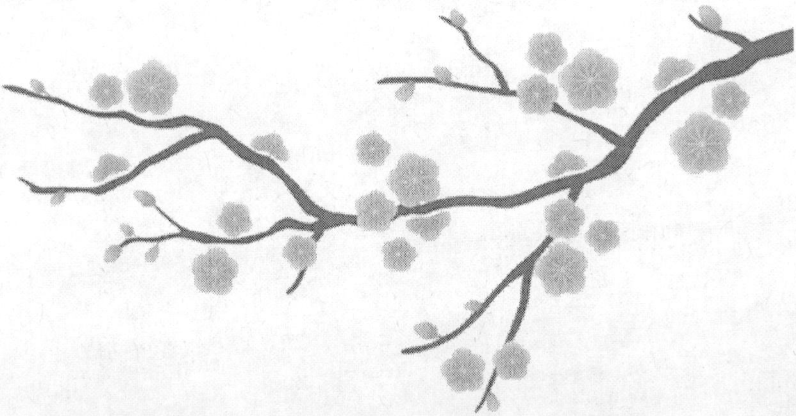

心